POCKET GUIDE TO
AROMATHERAPY

KATHI KEVILLE

THE CROSSING PRESS
FREEDOM, CALIFORNIA

I dedicate this book to everyone who has ever smelled a flower, sniffed the first scent of spring in the air or walked down the fragrant path of an herb garden. May your lives always be filled with fragrance!

Thank you to all the modern pioneers of aromatherapy who have brought this ancient art to the attention of the world. Thank you especially to aromatherapist Mindy Green, my friend and co-author of Aromatherapy *, The Fragrant Art of Healing. Her knowledge and inspiration are reflected in this pocket guide.*

CONTENTS

For an in depth coverage of Aromatherpy,
see
Aromatherapy:
A Complete Guide to the Healing Art.
By Kathi Keville and Mindy Green,
$16.95

What Is Aromatherapy?

"Aromatherapy" describes the use of essential oils—potent aromatic substances extracted from all fragrant plants—for physical and emotional healing. Today many herbalists, body workers, cosmetologists, chiropractors, and other holistic healers are discovering how this multifaceted and versatile healing art is able to enrich their practice. Many home healers as well are using the principles and resources of aromatherapy to expand their repertoire of natural remedies.

There are many approaches to using essential oils. Applied externally, they penetrate through the skin and are deposited in the underlying tissues. They also reach the bloodstream rather quickly: compounds from lavender oil have been detected in the blood only twenty minutes after the oil was rubbed on the skin.

As a result, one can treat a wide range of physical problems with aromatherapy. For example, massaging the appropriate aromatherapy body oil directly over the abdomen will quickly banish indigestion. Rubbing an aromatic vapor balm on the chest will relieve lung congestion and fight infection in two ways—as an inhalant drawn deep into the lungs' air passages, and as a lotion that penetrates the skin. Aromatherapy cosmetics and skin preparations are also used to counter external problems such as skin infections and eczema.

Interest in the therapeutic effects of inhaling essential oils continues to grow. More and more commonly, fragrances are being pumped into offices, stores, and even some hospitals to make the atmosphere more relaxing. Large corporations are turning to other fragrances to keep their workers alert, and more content, on the job. Inhaling certain essential oils has even been shown to lower blood pressure.

The beauty of aromatherapy is that you can take advantage of its physical and emotional applications in the same treatment. For example, you can blend a combination of essential oils that will not only stop indigestion, but calm you down and reduce the nervous condition that led to the indigestion. Or, you can design an aromatherapy body lotion that will not only improve your complexion, but relieve depression.

In the pages that follow, I will describe all of these methods and more, providing plenty of recipes along the way to get you started. I will also be looking into the cosmetic applications of aromatherapy in skin and hair-care products. If I succeed in sparking your interest in aromatherapy, be sure to have a look at the book I wrote last year with Mindy Green, *Aromatherapy: The Complete Guide to the Healing Art* (also from The Crossing Press), which goes into greater detail about using essential oils and making your own aromatherapy products.

Questions Most Frequently Asked About Aromatherapy

Is aromatherapy a new science?

Aromatherapy goes back to at least 4000 B.C., when Neolithic ointments combined vegetable oils with aromatic plants. Throughout the world, cultures began using aromatic steams, smoke, and water for healing. By around 3000 B.C., the uses of odoriferous herbs were being recorded on papyrus by the Egyptians, and on clay tablets in Mesopotamia and Babylonia. By 1700 B.C., trade routes had been established throughout the Middle East, mostly to permit traffic in solid aromatic unguents such as myrrh for incense, perfume and medicine, and aromatic spices for food. Eventually these routes extended into India, China, and Europe.

Essential oils were being distilled in Europe, China, and Japan by about 500 A.D., which led to the development of colognes, perfume, and facial waters. These were not only used to disguise body odor and improve the complexion, but were also ingested as medicinal tonics.

Appropriately, the birth of modern aromatherapy took place in France, the modern capital of perfume. It was Rene-Maurice Gattefossé, a French chemist descended from a long line of perfumers, who reunited the arts of perfumery and medicine. He coined the term "aromatherapy" around 1928 when a laboratory explosion in his family's perfume factory severely burned his hand. After plunging his injured hand into a container of lavender essential oil, he was amazed how quickly it healed. Young Gattefossé began to look for an answer.

Eventually Gattefossé's writings inspired others to explore aromatherapy, and interest in the new science spread to Europe and, finally, to the United States. Of course, most herbalists were already using aromatic plants in their healing work.

How is aromatherapy connected to herbalism?

Aromatherapy always has been a part of herbalism. The ancient Egyptians, Arabs, Greeks, Romans, and European herbalists all referred in their writings to the use of fragrance for healing purposes.

If you have ever used herbs, the chances are you have also experienced aromatherapy. Aromatic molecules, called essential oils, occur in any fragrant plant. Whenever you make a tea of, say, peppermint or chamomile, the heat draws essential oils from the plant into the water. You receive the healing benefits of essential oils both as you drink the tea and as you inhale the aroma. It is also possible to extract essential oils directly from herbs into alcohol or warm vegetable oil. (If you have an herb garden or other good supply of fragrant herbs, you may want to experiment.)

Aromatherapy differs from herbalism inasmuch as it employs only *certain* herbs. I like to think of it as a division of herbalism—one that uses fragrant plants exclusively. While non-fragrant herbs such as comfrey or goldenseal are not used in aromatherapy, many common medicinal herbs, such as elecampane, angelica, hyssop, and myrrh, are used, as are fragrant plants that are usually not considered medicinal, but do produce therapeutic essential oils. (Examples include ylang-ylang, vanilla, and mimosa.) Because herbs often contain several different types of medicinal compounds besides essential oils, herb books describing a fragrant herb's properties may not always be referring to properties associated with the essential oil.

What are essential oils?

Essential oils consist of tiny aromatic molecules that are released from a plant when you rub it, or just from the heat of hot summer day. (This is what makes an herb garden smell so fragrant.) Each type of essential oil is composed of many different aromatic molecules—more than 30,000 have been identified and named, and it is common for a single essential oil to contain one hundred different aromatic molecules.

The vast number of possible combinations of these molecules accounts for there being so many unique plant fragrances. However, because identical or very similar molecules occur in more than one plant, some plants smell very much alike, even when the plants in question are completely unrelated. This is especially true of the variety of plants that produce a lemon-like aroma; they include lemon itself, lemon verbena, melissa (lemon balm), lemon thyme, lemon eucalyptus, citronella, and palma rosa. Even though all of these plants and their corresponding essential oils smell similar, each one possesses a slightly different combination of aromatic molecules and carries its own distinctive olfactory shading.

In a few cases, a plant's essential oil is composed chiefly of one type of molecule. For example, sandalwood may contain up to 90 percent santalol, and clove bud has between 70 percent and 80 percent eugenol.

Why do plants produce essential oils?

At first, botanists were not sure why plants contain essential oils, which they viewed as mere by-products of plant metabolism. They were at a loss to explain why some plants produce essential oils and others do not, or why the fragrances vary so much from one plant to another.

Although there is still much to learn about why plants are fragrant, modern botanical research now understands that even though plants discard essential oils as waste products, the oils do serve important functions. Fragrances attract the insects that help to fertilize their flowers. They also protect plants by repelling certain insects, along with other predators. Many essential oils contain substances called terpenes, which help to waterproof the plant and protect it from rain. (Terpenes also make it difficult for many essential oils to mix with water.) Some essential oils are highly antiseptic, preventing the growth of bacteria, mold, and fungus on a plant.

How are essential oils obtained from plants?

The pure essential oils available at the local herb shop are usually extracted from plants through a process called steam distillation. Freshly picked plants are suspended over boiling water, with the steam drawing the oils out of the plant. The next step is to rapidly cool the steam back into water. During this process, the essential oil separates from the water.

There are several other ways to produce essential oils. One method squeezes, or presses, essential oils from the plant. Another very old method, rarely used today, is enfleurage, which extracts the oils into sheets of warm fat. Although various solvents may be used to extract essential oils, aromatherapists worry about the possibility of slight traces of the solvent contaminating the oils.

New methods of obtaining essential oils are currently being developed and introduced. One of the most interesting processes, although an expensive one, extracts the oil with carbon dioxide. The resulting essential oils have an odor very much like that of the original plant.

Can I make my own essential oils?

You can indeed make essential oils at home—but don't expect to produce very much! (It isn't unusual to obtain just a small vial of essential oil from a wheelbarrow full of plants.) The process is simple enough, although even a small commercial steam distiller costs several hundred dollars. You can also have a steam distiller custom-built by someone who does laboratory-glass blowing. Check the yellow pages for a chemistry supply house.

There is, however, a much cheaper way to rig up a home steam distiller in your kitchen, although you'll end up with even less essential oil than from a laboratory distiller. At the very least, you will obtain some excellent aromatic waters—and may even produce a few drops of oil. (For this reason, try distilling plants that yield a lot of oil, such as eucalyptus, rosemary, and peppermint.) Whether you purchase a distiller or rig one up at home, you will need to have a large supply of fresh plants because they release oil better and so much oil is lost when plants are dried.

To make an oil distiller at home, suspend a vegetable steamer full of fragrant herbs over a few inches of water in a pressure cooker. Place the pressure cooker on an unlit stove burner. Fasten the lid on the pressure cooker and attach the end of about six feet of plastic hose to the spout at the top. Coil the rest of the plastic tube in a bucket of ice water so that the tube's other end hangs outside the bucket. Stick this end of the tube into a quart-sized glass jar. For gravity to work, the bucket needs to stand below the pressure cooker, and the end of the tube needs to reach below the bottom of the bucket. Turn on the stove and boil the water in the pressure cooker. The steam will come out the spout and travel through the tube. When it hits the cold water, the oil and water will separate and pour together into the glass jar. The essential oil, which floats on top of the water, can be skimmed off. The resulting water (or "hydrosol") will also contain some essential oil.

Why are some essential oils so much more expensive than others?
The broad price range of essential oils—they vary from about $5 to $800 per ounce—reflects the range of difficulty involved in producing various oils. It is no wonder that Bulgarian rose oil sells for $600 an ounce—it took about six hundred pounds of rose petals to produce that ounce! On the other hand, plants such as eucalyptus and rosemary yield a comparatively large amount of essential oil, placing them among the least expensive.

There are several other reasons why it may be more expensive to produce one oil than another, including difficult growing conditions and the relative scarcity of certain plants. For example, peppermint is relatively easy to cultivate and propagate, and is harvested with machinery. Compare that to roses, which must be carefully cultivated, pruned, and hand-harvested.

Another consideration is the country in which the plant is grown. Peppermint would be even less expensive than it is if most of it weren't grown in the United States, where labor and other production costs are high. Many herbs used for essential-oil production come from developing nations.

How does fragrance affect emotions?

When your olfactory sensors detect a particular aroma, this information is sent to areas of the brain that influence memory, learning, emotions, hormone balance, and even more basic survival mechanisms. Exactly how the brain processes this data is not completely understood, but we do know that certain fragrances act on the brain's primitive limbic system, also known as the "smell brain."

Researchers studying aromacology—the science of medicinal aromas—have discovered that exposure to some aromatic substances results in an alteration of brain waves. They suspect that aromas may work on the brain in still other ways. The fragrance research company International Fragrance and Flavor (IFF) has tested over two thousand subjects to better understand how certain scents relieve pain, call up deep-seated memories, and affect personality, behavior, and sleep patterns.

It is probably no surprise that many psychologists have incorporated aromatherapy into their practices. In the early 1920s, Italian psychologists Giovanni Gatti and Renato Cayola concluded that "the sense of smell has...an enormous influence on the function of the central nervous system." They used certain scents to sedate their patients, others as stimulants. In France, psychologist Jean Valnet uses vanilla to help his patients unlock childhood memories. Several large Tokyo corporations have followed the advice of staff psychologists and begun to circulate lemon, peppermint, and cypress through their air-conditioning systems to keep workers attentive—and reduce the urge to smoke. Aroma is also assisting truck drivers, railroad engineers, air traffic controllers, and others whose jobs require that they remain alert.

Yet another way that fragrance can affect emotion is through association. Psychologists have successfully helped people overcome anxiety and other emotional problems by first inducing a state of relaxation, often with pleasant music, then introducing a strong scent. After several exposures to the scent, the patients begin to associate it with a tranquil state. The patients are then encouraged to carry vials of that scent out into the world, and whenever they encounter a situation that makes them tense, nervous or anxious, open the bottle, sniff, and relax.

Why are so many cosmetologists working with aromatherapy?

The answer to why aromatherapy is becoming so important to so many cosmetics firms—including Revlon, Redkin, Avon, Charles of the Ritz, and the Japanese firm Shiseido—is easy: aromatherapy offers a complete health and beauty package for both skin and hair.

Actually, this is nothing new. Fragrant herbs have long been used to clear complexions and make hair silky. Certain essential oils stimulate oil production in dry skin and hair. Others slow down overactive oil glands. Still others soothe and heal irritated skin. Many cosmetics firms now add botanical derivatives in order to cash in on the popularity of natural ingredients. Be sure to read the labels carefully and thoroughly when choosing skin-care products, and remember that you, too, can make aromatherapy body-care products, for only a fraction of what you would pay at the store (*see Creating Formulas*, page 18).

Can I learn to like scents that bother me at first?

I know several people who, consciously or unconsciously, have felt uncomfortable with, or even disliked, a person because he or she wears the same fragrance as someone with whom they once had problems. I met one man who hated the smell of lavender because the funeral parlor in his home-town had used it. Many people in his family had died when he was young, and, as a result, he had come to associate lavender with death and grief.

It takes time to change a negative reaction to a fragrance, although usually not all that much work. When you are in a good mood or in a place you enjoy, sniff a faint amount of the problematic scent combined with another scent, one that you do like. After doing this several times, you should begin to associate the once-disliked fragrance with pleasant experiences. (If this doesn't work, don't despair—aromatherapy offers so many different and appealing fragrances, you can afford to let one go.)

Creating Formulas

GETTING STARTED

Making and using aromatherapy products for healing or skin-care is not all that difficult. Some basic information about essential oils and a few safety tips are all you need to conduct your first experiments. Start with simple remedies and a few essential oils. As you become more familiar with the fragrances and properties of the different oils, the process will become easier and easier. For specific therapeutic and cosmetic applications, you can follow the suggestions in the five chapters following this one (pages 29-75) for your first experiments, or take inspiration from the descriptions of individual oils in the *Materia Medica*, page 78. Be sure to take careful notes so that you can duplicate a success—or avoid repeating a flop.

The most effective aromatherapy preparations have a fragrance so subtle you can barely perceive it. Use your nose as your guide, and don't be afraid to experiment. Most people prefer familiar and enjoyable fragrances. Remember, however, that not everyone likes the same fragrances. No matter how many books say that lavender is relaxing and promotes smiling, if you associate that fragrance with a bad memory, you may never learn to enjoy it.

EQUIPMENT

Unless you plan to extract your own essential oils, you will need very little equipment to make aromatherapy preparations at home. You probably have almost everything you need already in your kitchen. Vegetable oils such as almond, apricot, grape seed, and jojoba are available in most natural-food stores. The glass droppers you will need to measure out small amounts of the essential oils and transfer them from bottle to bottle are sold in drug stores, and in some natural-food stores. (While it is important not to contaminate your essential oils by moving the dropper directly from one vial of oil to the next, you don't need to have a separate dropper for each oil. Simply rinse the oily dropper in rubbing alcohol and wait a few minutes for the alcohol to completely evaporate before putting the dropper into another bottle.)

If you prefer, you may also use a narrow glass tube called a "pipette"—sold in chemical-equipment catalogs, in some drug stores, and on the pages of aromatherapy supply catalogs—to measure out small amounts of essential oils. Place one end in the essential oil, the other in your mouth. Gently inhale to draw the essential oil slowly up the tube. Well before it reaches the top of the tube, put your finger over the end you had in your mouth and move the pipette to another bottle. Every time you raise your finger, a little bit of oil will drop out. The most useful pipettes have graduated markings along the side so you can measure out exactly the amount of oil you wish to use.

Supply Checklist

Essential oils (see below)
Carrier—vegetable oils (see below), glycerin, distilled
        water, vodka or grain alcohol
Pyrex measuring cup
Clean, empty glass bottles with lids
Set of measuring spoons
Glass droppers (or pipettes)
Small funnel (optional)
Notebook, pencil, labels for bottles

Clean-up supplies:
>   paper towels
>   rubbing alcohol

Essential Oil Starter Kit

Besides a few pieces of equipment that you probably already have in your kitchen, you will need a few essential oils. These are sold at many natural-food stores and herb stores, as well as in mail-order catalogs (see *Resources*, page 102). For a starter kit, I recommend the following oils:

Lavender—fights infection, inflammation, insomnia, pain, depression, anxiety.

Chamomile—digestive and relaxation aid; treats allergies, rashes, menstrual cramps, inflammation, anxiety, anger, and depression.

Rosemary—relieves pain, congestion, constipation, and grief; stimulates circulation and memory; helps in times of transition.

Tea tree—fights most types of infection.

Peppermint—relieves indigestion, sinus congestion, itching, panic; mental stimulant.

Lemon (or other citrus)—antidepressant; kills parasites; promotes a sense of sense of cleanliness.

Geranium—balances mind and body.

Popular Carrier Oils

Almond	Coconut	Olive
Apricot	Grape seed	Rice Bran
Avocado	Hazelnut	Safflower
Canola	Jojoba	Sesame
Castor	Kukui	Squalene
Corn	Macadamia	

MEDIA

The most technologically refined way to fragrance a room is with an electric aromatic diffuser (see *Glossary*, page 97). You can also scent a room by placing a few drops of essential oil into a pan of water that is gently steaming on the stove, or into a small amount of water in a potpourri cooker. You can use these methods to change the room's emotional atmosphere, or to prevent airborne bacteria from spreading infection throughout your house. Another way to scent a room is with a drop or two of essential oil on a special ring designed to rest over a hot light bulb. Scented pillows, bed linens, clothes, and stationery are also common aromatherapy media.

Essential oils are often diluted in carrier oils (see list above). Most aromatherapy applications are two percent (two drops essential oil per one hundred drops carrier oil). A one-percent dilution is better for children, pregnant women, and those with particular health concerns. Some people find it easier to measure in drops, or in teaspoons, which are more convenient for large quantities. As mentioned earlier, a drug-store dropper is usually accurate enough, although the size of drops will vary depending on the size of the dropper opening, the temperature, and the viscosity (thickness) of the essential oil. See *Dilutions and Doses*, page 99, for information on diluting different types of aromatherapy preparations.

TIPS ON CREATING CUSTOM FORMULAS

The many choices that go into the creation of a blend may seem intimidating at first, but they also add to the excitement. Remember to keep records of how you make your preparations; include ingredients, proportions, processing procedures, and comments. Label your finished products with the ingredients, date, and any special instructions. When combining essential oils in a therapeutic blend, it is best for a beginner to use no more than five oils at a time. That way you will avoid unpredictable results due to the complex chemistries involved. Don't worry—you can create a safe and effective remedy with even one or two oils.

You may wish to take a few hints from professional perfumers. Think of each oil as having a unique personality. In the perfume trade, the "top note," "middle note," and "low note" define an essential oil's evaporation rate. Fragrances that are light and airy, like lavender, are top notes. Those that are heavy and linger—patchouli and vetiver, for example—are low notes. The middle notes lie somewhere in between. Carefully developed perfume blends that contain all three notes; beginners will especially want to avoid blends of exclusively pungent, heavy low notes.

Essential oils vary in odor intensity, and you will need to add much smaller amounts of some oils to your blends than others. You can tell the oils with a high odor intensity—such as chamomile, patchouli, cinnamon, ylang-ylang, and clary sage—just by smelling them.

If all this talk about "high notes," "middle notes," "low notes," and "intensity" is beginning to make you nervous, here are a few shortcuts for beginning aromatherapists. You can start with an essential oil that has a fairly complex chemistry and already smells like a blend; try geranium, which contains hints of herbs, rose, pine, cedar, and lemon. You can then expand your formula by adding small amounts of other oils, one at a time. When in doubt, choose one of the fragrances that already exists in the complex oil. With geranium, that could be cedarwood, sandalwood, or a citrus such as bergamot or petitgrain.

Another interesting way to expand a blend is to choose oils that are similar to each other. This performs a delightful trick on the nose when the oils begin to play off one another, making your blend seem more complicated and mysterious than it actually is. Try combining peppermint and spearmint, lemon and bergamot, or cinnamon and ginger. Every choice you make will take your blend in a new and interesting direction.

INCORPORATING HERBS

When used together, herbs and essential oils possess a greater capacity for healing than either on its own. Oils made by soaking herbs in vegetable oil are called "infused oils" and may be used in place of plain vegetable oil in aromatherapy preparations, resulting in more potent medicines. You can also add essential oils to salves, lotions, and creams to enhance their healing properties.

REGARDING QUALITY

To make a quality product, you will need to start with quality essential oils. Factors determining quality include purity, growing conditions, differences among species, and extraction techniques.

Purity is of concern to anyone purchasing essential oils. Rare and expensive oils are the most likely candidates for adulteration, and it is often difficult for an untrained nose to tell the difference between expensive pure essential oil of lemon verbena or melissa, and those same oils mixed with cheap lemongrass or citronella. (In fact, these oils are so often adulterated, you may never have smelled the real thing.) An essential oil that is cut with another oil will not necessarily carry the same properties, and certainly won't smell the same.

At first, it may seem difficult to judge quality, and unfortunately, store clerks do not always know a lot about aromatherapy and essential oils. Like many people, they think that anything marked "essential oil" is pure and natural. Enter the store armed with a little knowledge, and don't be shy about asking questions. You should be able to tell quickly whether the staff person is knowledgeable about essential oils. Some of the best aromatherapy companies are those run by aromatherapists, who are staking their reputations on supplying good essential oils. See *Resources*, page 101, for information on mail-ordering.

Quality can vary greatly due to climate and botanical differences. A good example is lavender, available in about a dozen different grades. There is often variation even within the grades, according to where the oil comes from and the year of harvest. Many commercial sources sell the least expensive grades of essential oil so they can offer them at a competitive price.

You don't always need to use the highest grade of essential oil, but you should at least know what you are buying. Go into a store that offers essential oils from several different companies and see if you can't smell the difference. The higher-grade essential oils generally carry more of a bouquet, a fuller-bodied fragrance.

The less expensive oils can cost more in the long run. A woman I know who makes facial creams had to use four times as much essential oil to achieve the same results when she switched to an inferior grade. Also, the fact that one essential oil smells different from another doesn't always mean that one of them is an inferior product. Sometimes variations exist in oils of comparable quality; in such cases, personal preference is your only guide.

A common method of adulterating essential oils is by "extending" (i.e., diluting) them with vegetable oils, alcohol, or some other solvent. One way to tell if an oil has been diluted with vegetable oil is to put a small drop on a piece of paper. Because they are so volatile, most essential oils will evaporate rather quickly, leaving no residue, and unless you are using very dark oils such as patchouli or benzoin, or a brightly colored oil such as German chamomile, no discoloration should remain. (Even with thick or colored oils, the stain should not be oily.)

While oils diluted with alcohol can be detected by a slight "boozy" odor, it is much harder to tell when the oil has been diluted with other clear, non-oily solvents. This is a potentially dangerous situation, because such solvents are readily absorbed into the body when rubbed on the skin or inhaled through the lungs. In such cases, you may have to rely on training your nose. Once you have experienced the intensity of an undiluted essential oil, oils cut with a solvent or synthetic just won't smell as good.

Problems with Synthetic Oils

When I pass around high-quality essential oils in my aromatherapy seminars, I warn my students that I am about to spoil them for life. Once you have smelled the real thing, it is difficult to use anything else. Synthetics, usually made with petroleum-based chemicals, try to duplicate natural scents; in my opinion, they never come close. They also are potentially harmful, since their tiny molecules penetrate the skin and enter the bloodstream.

Sad to say, synthetic fragrances permeate our lives. Many body-care products sold in natural-food stores contain them. Most fruits and flowers oils do not naturally produce essential oils, so when you see "essential oil" of carnation, lily of the valley, strawberry, or gardenia, you can be sure these are synthetics. When someone says that they react adversely or are allergic to fragrances, I am always suspicious. The chances are they have encountered only synthetics.

Proper Storage

Once you've gone to the trouble of locating and purchasing quality essential oils, you will want to keep them that way. Store them in glass vials with tight lids in a cool place. The glass may be clear instead of amber, but remember to keep essential oil out of direct sunlight.

Properly stored, most essentials oil will keep for years. Citrus oils, such as orange and lemon, are the most vulnerable to oxidation and spoilage, but even they will last a couple of years if refrigerated. A few essential oils, such as patchouli, clary sage, benzoin, vetiver, and sandalwood, actually improve with age. (I have some twenty-year-old patchouli that smells so rich, people have trouble identifying the fragrance—even those who normally hate the smell of patchouli.)

I store even diluted aromatherapy products in glass. Pure essential oils stored in plastic, or in bottles with plastic droppers, will eventually eat away the plastic. The obvious danger is that the oil will leak out of the container, but long before that occurs, the oil will have been contaminated. There are times, however, when glass can weigh you down. Say you want a lightweight first-aid kit or a toiletries case for traveling, or maybe you just want to carry a lotion or cream down to the beach or up onto the ski slopes. It is safe to temporarily store essential oils and products containing essential oils in plastic containers—just be sure that the containers are made of a durable, stiff grade of plastic.

SAFETY

—Overexposure to essential oils, either through the skin or by nose, can result in nausea, headache, skin irritation, emotional unease, or an overall "spaced out" feeling. Getting some fresh air will help you to overcome these symptoms.

—To use an essential oil internally, your best bet is to take the herb as a tea or a tincture.

—Essential oils are very potent, concentrated substances, capable, if undiluted, of burning or irritating skin and other sensitive tissues. Keep all essential oils away from mucous membranes (the lining of the digestive, respiratory, and genito-urinary tracts) and eyes. If you ever experience skin irritation from contact with essential oils, or accidentally get some in the eyes, flush with straight vegetable oil, not water.

Potential Skin Irritants

bay rum	citronella	thyme (except
birch	clove	type linalol)
black pepper	cumin	thuja
cinnamon		

—Use essential oils cautiously with anyone who is elderly, convalescing, or who has a serious health problem such as asthma, epilepsy, or heart disease. If there is any chance a person may be sensitive or allergic to an essential oil, run a patch test, placing

27

one drop of the suspect essential oil in one-quarter teaspoon of vegetable oil and rubbing a little of the mixture into the crook of the arm or the back of the neck at the hairline. Wait twelve hours to see if a reaction occurs.

—Certain essential oils cause a photosensitizing reaction that produces an uneven pigmentation on the skin, so use them with caution—and never in a suntan lotion. The most notorious such oil is bergamot, which contains bergaptene, a powerful photosensitizer.

Photosensitizing Essential Oils

angelica	cumin (slightly)	lime (slightly)
bitter orange	lemon (slightly)	orange (slightly)

—Vary the essential oils you use. Uninterrupted use of some oils exposes your liver and kidneys to chemical constituents that may be harmful over time.

POTENTIALLY TOXIC ESSENTIAL OILS

The following oils are not included in the Materia Medica, which begins on page 75. *NEVER* administer these oils to children or pregnant women:

bitter almond (*Prunus amygdalus*, var. *Amara*)
hyssop (*Hyssopus officinalis*)
mugwort (*Artemesia vulgaris*)
oregano (*Origanum vulgare*)
pennyroyal (*Mentha pelugium*)
sassafras (*Sassafras albidum*)
savory (*Satureja hortensis*)
thuja (*Thuja occidentalis*)

Aromatherapy and Emotional Health

How aroma effects the mind is not completely understood, although we do know that when you smell something, information is sent to the specific areas of the brain that influence memory, learning, emotions, hormone balance, and even basic survival mechanisms such as the fight-or-flight response. Psychologists have begun working with fragrances to enhance interaction and communication among people. Pleasant smells seem to make people more willing to negotiate, cooperate, and compromise with others.

The formulas in this section can be used as body, massage, or bath oils. If you are a health-care practitioner, one subtle way in which to practice aromatherapy with your patients is to dab a small amount of an appropriate essential oil on the back of your hand. If you would rather scent the room, use the essential oils suggested in the following formulas in a diffuser, a potpourri cooker, a pan of simmering water, or on a light-bulb ring.

DEPRESSION

Certain fragrances affect brain waves in a fashion similar to antidepressant drugs, according to research by the Olfaction Research Group at Warwick University in England. At his clinic in France, psychologist Paolo Rovesti has successfully pulled many patients out of depression with the citrus scents of orange, bergamot, lemon, and lemon verbena. One of my favorite aromatic antidepressants, the elegant scent of neroli essential oil, is also a citrus. Sixteenth-century herbalist

John Gerard said that melissa "gladdens the heart" and that clary sage counters depression, paranoia, mental fatigue, and nervous disorders. Other antidepressant essential oils include jasmine, sandalwood, and ylang-ylang.

Anti-depressive Essential Oils

bergamot	lavender	orange
clary sage	lemon	petitgrain
geranium	lemon verbena	sandalwood
grapefruit	melissa	tangerine
jasmine	neroli	ylang-ylang

Anti-depressive Formula

12 drops bergamot
6 drops petitgrain
6 drops rose geranium
1 drop neroli (expensive, so optional)
4 ounces vegetable oil

Combine ingredients.

ANXIETY

Aromatherapists use several fragrances to help overcome feelings of anxiety, loneliness, and rejection. I find the same oils useful for anyone undergoing a major life transition.

Anxiety-relieving Essential Oils

basil	hyssop	orange
bergamot	lavender	rose
cedarwood	marjoram	
cypress	opopanax	
	(similar to myrrh)	

Anxiety Formula

12 drops lavender
6 drops orange
3 drops marjoram
3 drops cedarwood
4 ounces vegetable oil

Combine ingredients.

FATIGUE

A Japanese alarm clock manufacturer has designed an apparatus that uses eucalyptus and pine to awaken sleepers. Throughout the workday, lemon, cypress, and peppermint circulate through the air-conditioning systems of several large Tokyo companies to keep employees alert. The spicy aromas of clove, basil, black pepper, cinnamon, and, to a lesser degree, patchouli, lemongrass, and sage are known to reduce drowsiness, irritability, and headaches. Instead of over-amping the adrenal glands with caffeine and other stimulants, these oils actually counteract the rush of adrenaline. They also prevent the sharp drop in attention typical after thirty minutes of work. In Italy, doctors Giovanni Gatti and Renato Cayola use clove, cinnamon, lemon, ylang-ylang, cardamom, fennel, and angelica to stimulate patients.

Stimulating Essential Oils

angelica	cinnamon	lemon
basil	clove	peppermint
benzoin	cypress	pine
black pepper	eucalyptus	
camphor	fennel	

Stimulant Formula

15 drops lemon
4 drops eucalyptus
3 drops peppermint
1 drops cinnamon
1 drop benzoin (optional)
4 ounces vegetable oil

Combine ingredients.

MEMORY

Researchers have learned that mental recall improves dramatically when a past event is associated with smell. That's why a whiff of a perfume or other fragrance can send you back in time, evoking long-forgotten images and feelings. Next to my computer, I keep a sprig of rosemary, whose ability to increase memory, concentration, and even creativity is legendary. Modern Japanese research confirms that rosemary is a brain stimulant. Other mental stimulants include sage, basil, and bay leaf.

Memory-stimulating Essential Oils

bay	lavender	rosemary
jasmine	lemon	

Memory Formula

10 drops lavender
8 drops lemon
5 drops rosemary
1 drop cinnamon
4 ounces vegetable oil

Combine ingredients.

GRIEF

In the sixteenth century, herbalist John Gerard wrote that basil "taketh away sorrowfulness…and maketh a man merry and glad" and suggested a whiff of marjoram "for those given to much sighing" from grief, loneliness, or rejection. Ancient Egyptians, Greeks, and Romans also sniffed marjoram to "strengthen emotions" and mitigate grief. The Greeks used cypress and hyssop to comfort mourners; several ancient cultures burned sandalwood at death ceremonies to accomplish the same purpose. In Europe, sage, clary sage, and rosemary were used to overcome grief. These essential oils can also be used during a transition in one's life, such as a job change or the end of a romantic relationship. Other good companions include the gentle, relaxing scents of lavender and marjoram, both used traditionally to comfort the sick, the dying, and their families.

Essential Oils to Ease Grief

basil	fir	myrrh
clary sage	hyssop	rosemary
cypress	marjoram	sandalwood

Grief Formula
---

8 drops marjoram
6 drops melissa or lemon
4 drops clary sage
4 drops cypress or rosemary
1 drop hyssop essential oil
   (expensive, so optional)
4 ounces vegetable oil

Combine ingredients.

INSOMNIA

Lack of sleep is problem for millions of Americans, often leading to agitation, depression, dizziness, and headaches.

Essential Oils for Insomnia

bergamot	lavender	nutmeg
chamomile	lemon	patchouli
clary sage	marjoram	rose
frankincense	melissa	sandalwood
jasmine	myrrh	valerian
geranium	neroli	ylang-ylang

Insomnia Formula

12 drops bergamot
6 drops chamomile
5 drops geranium
1 drop frankincense
1 drop rose
4 ounces vegetable oil

Combine ingredients.

STRESS

Fragrances can lower your pulse and breathing rate. Place people in a room scented with lavender, bergamot, marjoram, sandalwood, lemon, or chamomile, and notice the reduction in avoidance and competition. In his seventeenth-century *Herbal*, Nicholas Culpeper agreed that chamomile "comforts" the head and brain. In more modern times, doctors Giovanni Gatti and Renato Cayola have found that the most sedating oils for their patients are neroli, petitgrain, chamomile, valerian, and opopanax.

International Flavors and Fragrance researchers have patented a blend of neroli, valerian, and nutmeg to ease stress in the workplace. Aromatherapists class ylang-ylang among the most potent of all aromatherapy relaxants.

Essential Oils to Reduce Stress

basil	jasmine	petitgrain
bergamot	lavender	rose
cardamom	marjoram	sandalwood
clove	melissa	valerian
chamomile	myrrh	vanilla
clary sage	neroli	ylang-ylang
frankincense	nutmeg	
helicrysum	orange	

Sedative Formula

8 drops lavender
4 drops sandalwood
4 drops bergamot
4 drops chamomile
3 drops ylang-ylang
2 drops petitgrain
4 ounces vegetable oil

Combine ingredients.

APHRODISIACS

Research tells us that many of the fragrances known traditionally as aphrodisiacs both stimulate and relax brain waves. Examples are ylang-ylang, rose, patchouli, sandalwood, and jasmine. Aphrodisiacs that are primarily stimulants include cinnamon and coriander (named as an aphrodisiac in *The Arabian Nights*). Both of these essential oils may also be used to relieve stress.

Aphrodisiac Oils

cinnamon	patchouli	vanilla
coriander	rose	ylang-ylang
jasmine	sandalwood	

Aphrodisiac Formula

12 drops sandalwood
5 drops ylang-ylang
5 drops vanilla
1 drop cinnamon
1 drop jasmine
4 ounces vegetable oil

Combine ingredients.

SPIRITUAL

Throughout the world, ancient cultures have regarded incense as a mediator between the worshippers and deity, a creator of ethereal roads along which prayers travel. Aromas that smell "heavenly" were acknowledged to have powers of purification; less pleasant odors were thought to bring on disease or death, or to cleanse the impure. A special reverence was given trees, for they seemed to join earth and sky (again, the mundane with the divine); their smoke, therefore, was used to communicate between these worlds. Sandalwood, the famous "cedars of Lebanon," Tibetan cedar, American cedar, juniper, cypress, and camphor were just a few of these holy trees whose sap was correlated with blood and took its place in ritual practices. Rosemary and marjoram were included because they represented both birth and death, and were used at both weddings and funerals. Lavender is still burned with heavier resins such as myrrh in some Greek Orthodox churches.

Spiritual Essential Oils

camphor	juniper	rosemary
cedar	lavender	sandalwood
cypress	marjoram	
frankincense	myrrh	

Spiritual Formula
---

8 drops sandalwood
8 drops cedarwood
6 drops lavender
2 drops frankincense
2 drops myrrh

Combine ingredients.

Aromatherapy and Skin Care

The techniques and the essential oils you choose for your overall skin care should be based on your complexion type. There are several different types of complexions, the most distinctive being dry and oily. There are is also a "mature" complexion (generally dry) and a "problem" complexion, associated with the kinds of conditions—such as blackheads and acne. A "couperose" complexion is sensitive skin that has fine red lines on the nose or cheeks; treat it according to whether it is oily or dry. (Essential oils that decrease inflammation will help to reduce the redness.) Many people fall into more than one skin-type category, and as a result need to be treated as though they possess two or more different complexions.

FACIAL TECHNIQUES SUITABLE FOR MOST COMPLEXION TYPES

A facial is one of the kindest things you can give your complexion. The complete treatment includes cleansing, steaming, exfoliation, and a mask, topped off with a facial toner or cream. All of these techniques increase circulation, giving your face a healthful and radiant glow. Exfoliation and steaming may be done once a week on complexions other than extremely dry or delicate skin (such as couperose). Delicate and dry complexions can use masks once a week, but stick to the gentler ones. Toners may be used as an all-over body treatment, as a facial, or as an after-shave.

Cleansing: Clean your face gently with cold cream or vegetable oil after removing any makeup.

Steaming: Besides cleansing and leaving your face looking youthful and vibrant, steaming moisturizes skin and unclogs pores.

Exfoliation: A gentle scrubbing that removes dead skin cells from the skin's surface, brings young, fresh skin to the surface, stimulates growth of underlying cells, and even gives the impression of diminishing wrinkles. Avoid the chemical exfoliants used in some beauty salons.

Mask: A facial mask absorbs, moisturizes, and may (depending upon the ingredients) remineralize the skin. Astringent masks of oats, cream of wheat, and clay also exfoliate the skin. Gentler masks include honey, avocado, egg whites, and fresh fruits such as papaya and yogurt. Adding the appropriate ground herbs will increase the skin-healing properties.

Toning: Astringent toners draw water from underlying skin levels to the surface, temporarily plumping it up and diminishing enlarged pores and wrinkles. They offer oily and "problem" skins a good alternative to oil-based moisturizers, and can double as a men's aftershave.

Facial Steam

> 5 drops lavender
> 5 drops rosemary
> 5 drops geranium
> One quart boiling water

Bring water to a simmer, remove from heat, and add essential oils. Holding your face about twelve inches above the pan, place the towel over the back of your head and tuck the ends around the pan to enclose your face in a miniature sauna. Be sure to keep your eyes closed so they won't be irritated by the essential oils. Steam for a few minutes, then remove your head and take a few breaths of fresh air. Go back under the towel and repeat a few times. (Steam for no longer than five or ten minutes per session, or less if you have sensitive skin.)

Facial Scrub

3 tablespoons oatmeal
1 tablespoon cornmeal
water, tea, or hydrosol to moisten

Grind ingredients in an electric-coffee grinder. Store powder in a closed container. To use the scrub, moisten one teaspoon with enough water, tea, or hydrosol to make a paste. Apply to a dampened face. Gently scrub and rinse with warm water.

Exfoliating Mask

1 tablespoon finely ground oats, or clay
1 teaspoon honey, slightly heated
1 drop carrot seed oil
1–2 teaspoons aloe vera juice (or herb tea)

Mash oats or clay into a thin paste with honey and aloe. Stir in essential oil. Apply to the face in an even layer, avoiding sensitive areas around eyes and mouth. Leave on 5–30 minutes, or as long as comfortable. (Don't allow the mask to dry or pull so much that it becomes irritating.) Finally, wash the mask off with warm water and gently pat the face dry.

DRY SKIN

Cleanser: Instead of soap, which is drying, use a water-soluble cleansing cream that won't remove natural skin oils. Do this no more than once per day. Gently pat skin dry.

Steaming: Restrict steaming to five minutes every other week.

Exfoliation: Gently massage face for two minutes with a gentle oatmeal scrub to stimulate oil production and exfoliate flaky, dry surface skin.

Mask: Moisturize with an emollient mask of honey, yogurt, avocados, or egg yolks. Avoid drying clay masks.

Toning: Moisturize with a cream, a toner made with aloe vera, or a hydrosol to increases water content. Diluted apple-cider vinegar relieves the itching and flakiness of dry skin. Avoid alcohol, which is too drying.

Moisturizing: Use rich facial creams, and make-ups that contain moisturizers.

Essential Oils for Dry Skin

The following oils balance skin-oil production, and most reduce puffiness and rejuvenate skin by encouraging new cell growth. If your dry skin is also mature skin, use the classic "anti-aging" ingredients: lavender, geranium, neroli, rosemary, and rose.

carrot seed	jasmine	rosemary
chamomile	lavender	(especially the
cistus	myrrh	chemotype
frankincense	neroli	verbenone)
geranium	palmarosa	rosewood
helichrysum	peppermint	sandalwood

Dry-complexion Cleanser

8 drops sandalwood
4 drops rosemary
1/2 teaspoon grapefruit-seed extract
2 ounces aloe gel

> 1 teaspoon glycerin
> 1 teaspoon vegetable oil

Blend ingredients. Shake well before each use. Apply with cotton pads, then rinse off. I like to use an infused herb oil of calendula for the vegetable oil.

Dry-complexion Toner

> 6 drops geranium
> 4 drops sandalwood
> 1 drop chamomile
> 1 drop jasmine (optional)
> 800 IUs vitamin E oil
> 2 ounces aloe vera gel
> 2 ounces orange blossom water
> 1 teaspoon vinegar

Combine ingredients. Shake before using. To obtain liquid vitamin E oil, you may pop open a couple of 400 IU vitamin E gel capsules. Jasmine is "optional" only because it is so expensive.

OILY SKIN

Cleanser: Clean at least twice a day with a neutral pH soap, or with cleansing gel and water.

Steaming: Steam weekly to unclog pores and release excess oil.

Exfoliation: Use a mild abrasive such as corn meal mixed with oatmeal, but don't scrub vigorously, which will stimulate oil production.

Mask: Both oats and clay draw excess skin oils, but be sure to rinse before skin begins to feel tight or itchy.

Toning: Aloe vera, hydrosols, and witch hazel improve the complexion without adding oil. Grain alcohol in a tincture such as witch hazel dries the skin, although too much will cause the skin to compensate by producing even more oil.

Moisturizing: Use a light lotion instead of a cream. Just a little oil will encourage the skin to cut down on its own oil production.

Essential Oils for Oily Skin

The following oils normalize overactive sebaceous glands, slowing oil production.

basil	cypress	sage
cedarwood	eucalyptus	spike lavender
citruses	lemongrass	ylang-ylang

Oily-skin Cleanser

1 teaspoon vinegar
1 teaspoon glycerin
1/2 teaspoon grapefruit seed extract
6 drops lemon
2 drops cypress
2 drops grapefruit (optional)
2 ounces witch hazel

Follow the instructions given above for dry-skin cleanser. If available, you can use an herbal vinegar. I make my own yarrow vinegar for this formula, but a basil or sage vinegar from the grocery store is fine.

Toner for Oily or "Problem" Complexion

5 drops cedarwood
3 drops lemon
1 drop ylang-ylang
1 tablespoon aloe vera
2 ounces witch hazel

Combine ingredients. Shake well before using. Without the ylang-ylang, which is too sweet-smelling for most men, this makes an excellent aftershave for men.

"PROBLEM" SKIN

Cleanser: Treat affected skin up to three times per day with a pH-balanced cleanser.

Steaming: Steam once or twice per week. Scrubbing and exfoliants only aggravate acne.

Mask: An astringent mask of clay mixed with antibacterial essential oils promotes peeling and reduces enlarged pores. A papaya mask will gently exfoliate.

Toning: Diluted cider vinegar is antiseptic and helps maintain the skin's acid balance. Antiseptic hydrosols or aloe vera (with its skin-healing properties and pH of 4.3) are excellent toners.

Moisturizing: Use light lotions containing mostly aloe vera.

Essential Oils for "Problem" Skin

The following oils are antiseptic and drying.

clary sage	rosemary	tea tree
eucalyptus	(especially	thyme
juniper	chemotype	(especially
lavender	verbenone)	chemotype
neroli	sage	linalol)

--- **Zit Remover** ---

4 drops lavender
1 teaspoon Epsom salts
1/4 cup water

Bring water to a boil and pour over salts. When the salts have dissolved, add the essential oil. Soak a small absorbent cloth in the solution and press this compress onto the pimple. In a minute or two, as it starts to cool, place the cloth back in hot water, then reapply. Repeat several times. The lavender is antiseptic and anti-inflammatory.

Intensive Treatment for Acne

> 12 drops tea tree
> 1/2 teaspoon goldenseal root, powdered
> water

Combine ingredients, adding water to create a paste. Apply directly onto acne spots. Let dry and remain on the skin for at least twenty minutes. Rinse.

FUNGAL AND VIRAL SKIN INFECTIONS

Aromatherapy offers many treatments against fungal and viral infections such as warts, herpes, and the related shingles virus, which causes the skin to break out in blisters along nerve endings. Treat these conditions externally by diluting an essential oil of tea tree, or with the closely related eucalyptus (especially lemon eucalyptus) in an equal amount of vegetable oil or alcohol and applying it directly to the blisters. Other excellent anti-viral and anti-fungal oils are lavender, myrrh, and geranium. If applied to herpes as soon as the blisters begin to appear, these oils will often prevent a break-out. Small amounts of peppermint relieve the itching of a fungal infection, and sometimes diminish the nerve-tingling pain of herpes and shingles.

Research shows that creams made from capsaicin, a compound found in cayenne, deadens the pain of herpes and shingles. Essential oils of cayenne will work if added to a cream or oil base, but be sure to go easy with it, since too much can burn the skin.

Use the same essential oils on skin warts, which are yet another type of virus. Tea tree and thuja are two of the most effective essential oils, even in cases of skin or genital warts. However, if genital warts don't begin to disappear in a few weeks or so, have a doctor remove them. The virus that causes them is passed onto sexual partners and can eventually lead to cervical dysplasia in women.

Many different types of fungal infections appear on the skin, but athlete's foot is the most common. A fungal powder (such as that described below) or plain vinegar provide the best base for a remedy to treat fungal infections. Both the powder and vinegar are drying.

Anti-fungal Powder

12 drops tea tree (or eucalyptus)
6 drops geranium
2 tablespoons bentonite clay

Drop essential oils into clay and mix well. Apply to the problem area. If you prefer a liquid formula, add these same ingredients to 1/2 cup apple-cider vinegar. A soft cloth soaked in the solution makes an excellent compress.

Wart Oil

12 drops tea tree
5 drops thuja
1/4 ounce castor oil
800 IU vitamin E oil

Combine ingredients. Apply two to four times per day with a glass rod or cotton swab to the warts only, since these essential oils can burn sensitive skin. If necessary, protect surrounding skin with a coating of herbal salve.

Herpes Formula

10 drops tea tree
(especially chemotype niaouli)
10 drops myrrh
4 drops geranium
1 ounce vodka

Apply to affected area at least two to three times per day.

BATHING

Bathing with essential oils is the ultimate aromatherapy treatment. The essential and vegetable oils float on the surface of the water and make your bath smell heavenly. When you emerge, the oils cling to your skin, scenting you for hours. Bath salts are another luxurious addition to your bath water, making the water feel silky, removing body oils and perspiration, softening the skin, relaxing the muscles, and soaking away the stresses of the day.

Floating Aromatic Bath Oil

1/2 teaspoon essential oil (your choice)
1 ounce vegetable oil

Combine ingredients. Use one teaspoon per bath. For babies, use only a few drops in the basin.

Aromatic Bath Salts

1/2 teaspoon essential oil (your choice)
1 cup sea salt
1/2 cup borax
1/2 cup baking soda

Mix salts together and add essential oils, mixing well to combine. Use 1/4 to 1/2 cup of the bath salts per bath. For muscular aches and pains, add 1/2 cup Epsom salts to this recipe. (All of the salts mentioned are sold in grocery stores.)

HAIR CARE

Whether you have dry, normal, or oily hair, essential oils have something to offer you. Besides making shampoos and hair rinses, you can run a couple drops of essential oil directly through the hair, which holds fragrance even better than skin, so you will remain fragrant for hours.

Oils for Dry Hair

cedarwood   rosewood   sandalwood

Oils for Oily Hair

cypress   lemongrass   patchouli

Oils for All Hair Types

chamomile   lavender   rosemary

Oils for Dandruff

cedarwood   sage   tea tree
geranium

Oils to Counteract Hair Loss

basil   peppermint   ylang-ylang
cedarwood

Herbal Shampoo

1/4 teaspoon essential oil (your choice)
2 ounces unscented shampoo
2 ounces strong herb tea (your choice)

After straining and cooling, add tea to the shampoo base, then add the essential oils. Shake well before using. Use a mild and pH-balanced shampoo as the base for this recipe. Baby shampoos, which are generally made from olive and soy oils, are a good choice.

Herbal Hair Rinse

3–5 drops essential oil (your choice)
1 pint of water or herb tea
4 tablespoons vinegar or lemon juice (optional)

Shake well and pour over the scalp and hair after shampooing. Leave on for several minutes, then rinse. This formula balances the pH after shampooing, reversing the electrical charge so your hair doesn't have a "fly-away" look, and removes shampoo residues, leaving hair shiny and soft.

Healing the Body with Aromatherapy

Most essential oils are germ-fighters, but their beneficial properties do not stop there. Essential oils can be digestive tonics, circulatory stimulants, or hormone precursors. Some oils even stimulate production of phagocytes, white blood cells that rid the body of pathogens. Fortunately, many essential oils perform more than one function, so you need only become familiar with a dozen or so to be able to tend to a wide range of common ailments.

When using aromatherapy to treat physical ailments, stick to simple disorders that you would self-diagnose and treat at home anyway, such as a minor sore throat or a bout of indigestion. Think of the remedies in this section as "over-the-counter" preparations. For more serious problems, be sure to seek the advice of a health professional, preferably one skilled in holistic healing and aromatherapy.

Although this section deals mostly with treating internal problems, essential oils are usually applied externally in a vegetable oil or alcohol base. Since the tiny molecules in essential oils are easily absorbed through the skin and into the bloodstream, external application concentrates them where they are needed. A massage oil blend designed to ease a stomach ache, for example, may be rubbed directly over the abdomen. It's also a good idea to also investigate complementary methods of healing—especially herbs, body work, diet, and lifestyle changes.

INCREASING IMMUNITY

Some of the same essential oils that are powerful antiseptics also encourage the immune system and increase the rate of healing. Many such oils fight infection by stimulating the production of white corpuscles, part of the body's immune defense. Still others encourage new cell growth to promote faster healing. All these oils can be used in conjunction with herbal remedies designed to increase immunity.

One important way to assist your immune system is with a lymphatic massage using essential oils in massage oil. The lymphatic system is responsible for moving cellular fluid through the system, cleansing the body of waste produced through the body's simple metabolic functions. Lymph nodes in the throat, groin, breasts, under the arms, and elsewhere are filtering centers for the blood. Among the best essential oils for the lymphatic system are true bay (*Laurus nobilis*), lemon, rosemary, and grapefruit. A lymphatic massage involves deep strokes that work from the extremities toward the heart. You can even massage yourself, rubbing the oil up your arms toward the lymph nodes in your armpits, and down your neck toward the chest.

Essential Oils for Immunity

cinnamon	lemon	tea tree
eucalyptus	oregano	thyme
lavender	sage	

Oils That Stimulate Production of White Corpuscles

bergamot	lemon	sandalwood
chamomile	myrrh	thyme
lavender	pine	vetiver

Oils That Encourage New Cell Growth

garlic   lavender   sandalwood

geranium   rose

Basic Immune Stimulant Blend

12 drops lavender
12 drops bergamot
5 drops tea tree
5 drops ravensare
5 drops caulophyllum inophyllum (if available)
4 ounces vegetable oil

Combine ingredients. Use as a general massage oil over areas of the body that tend to develop physical problems. For example, if you get a lot of chest colds and flus, rub this blend over your chest.

Lymph Massage Oil

12 drops lemon
12 drops rosemary
12 drops grapefruit
6 drops true bay *(Laurus nobilis)*
4 ounces vegetable oil

Combine ingredients.

INDIGESTION

The same essential oils that make food tasty help you digest the meals they flavor. Simply inhale the aromas of these herbs (see list below) and a signal is sent to the brain that begins a chain-reaction. Your stomach starts grumbling in anticipation as digestive fluids are pumped into the digestive tract to help you assimilate the approaching meal.

(Note: Smelling the essential oils of dill, and fennel may *decrease* the appetite.)

Putting essential oils that help digestion in a massage oil can help relieve belching, stomach pains, and intestinal gas. This is a particularly good treatment for young children or anyone who has trouble swallowing medicine. Some oils have special applications: cumin relieves headaches due to indigestion; rosemary improves poor food absorption; lemongrass relieves nervous indigestion; peppermint treats irritable-bowel syndrome. To overcome nausea, even from chemotherapy, try basil. Peppermint and ginger ease nausea and motion sickness. Chamomile, fennel, and melissa relax the stomach and soothe burning irritation and inflammation. Black pepper and juniper berry increase stomach acid; you can even sprinkle pepper on your meals, or chew a couple of juniper berries before eating, to obtain enough essential oil to do the trick.

General Digestive Aids

anise	cumin	oregano
basil	ginger	peppermint
chamomile	lemongrass	rosemary
cinnamon	melissa	thyme
coriander		

Digestive Massage Oil

12 drops orange
8 drops ginger
5 drops peppermint
3 drops fennel
4 ounces vegetable oil

Combine ingredients. Rub into abdomen. This all-purpose formula will help improve the appetite and digestion, and prevent nausea. (This formula can also be converted into a tea blend—see *Dilutions and Doses*, page 99 for proportions.)

Children's Bath for Indigestion

2 drops lemongrass
1 drop orange
1 drop chamomile

Add directly to bath water. Stir to distribute on the water's surface before getting into the tub.

INFECTIONS

Almost all essential oils are more or less antiseptic, destroying bacteria, fungi, yeast, parasites, and/or viruses. One way to use these essential oils for preventive medicine—even for internal infections—is in your bath. Another method is to rub a massage oil that contains them over the afflicted area. To treat a vaginal infection, douching brings the essential oils in direct contact with the yeast or bacteria that is causing the discomfort.

Bladder Infection Relief

8 drops tea tree
3 drops ravensare (if available)
3 drops fennel
1 ounce vegetable oil

Use as a massage oil applied over the kidney and bladder area two to three times per day. For a preventive treatment if you tend to get bladder infections, add a tablespoon of this oil to your bath.

Douche

> 3 drops lavender
> 3 drops tea tree
> 3 cups warm water
> 2 heaping tablespoons yogurt (optional)
> 3 cups water

Combine ingredients in a douche bag. Mix well. Use this douche once a day during an active infection. The yogurt helps establish the natural flora of the vagina and keeps the essential oils evenly distributed throughout the water. You can use these same essential oils, diluted in vegetable oil, as massage oil to rub on the abdomen, or add a few drops to a bath or a sitz bath.

MENOPAUSE

Several essential oils that contain hormone-like substances related to estrogen are advantageous during menopause. These include clary sage, anise, fennel, angelica, coriander, and sage. Geranium and lavender are reported to be hormonal balancers. They modify menopause symptoms and relieve hot flashes. One of the easiest ways to employ them is as a bath or body oil.

Menopause symptoms can also include a dry, less elastic vagina. An excellent essential oil to relieve this is neroli. A few drops can be added to a commercial cream—just stir it in with a toothpick—or you can blend the Rejuvenation Oil suggested below. If you buy a cream, choose one that is made with all-natural products.

In addition to these aromatherapy suggestions, seek out information on dietary and herbal treatments that may make menopause smoother.

Hormone Essential Oils

angelica	coriander	sage
anise	fennel	
clary sage	lavender and geranium (balancing)	

Menopause Body Oil

> 12 drops lemon
> 6 drops clary sage
> 6 drops peppermint (optional)
> 5 drops angelica
> 5 drops fennel
> 4 ounces vegetable oil

Combine ingredients. Use daily as a body oil. If this formula is too oily for you, add these same essential oils to four ounces of a commercial body lotion instead. The best type to use is an unscented, basic lotion with all-natural ingredients.

Rejuvenation Oil

> 6 drops rose geranium
> 6 drops lavender
> 1 drop neroli (expensive, and therefore optional)
> 1500 units vitamin E oil
> 1 ounces vegetable oil

Combine ingredients. (To obtain the vitamin E, either buy the liquid vitamin or open vitamin capsules and empty the contents.) Apply around and in the vagina as needed.

NERVE AND JOINT PAIN

Essential oils of lavender, helichrysum, chamomile, and marjoram are all specific for nerve pain. I know several people with serious problems related to the nervous system, such as multiple sclerosis and chronic fatigue syndrome, who get pain relief from the Nerve Pain Oil presented below. While it may not offer a cure, it can certainly improve the quality of life. For carpal tunnel syndrome, rub this oil into the wrists. Use it on the back or hip for a pinched nerve or sciatica, and on shingles (a painful skin eruption related to herpes) to reduce pain. For arthritis, rheumatism, and other inflammatory conditions, use chamomile, marjoram, birch, and ginger.

Nerve conditions can be difficult to heal, so talk to someone skilled in natural medicine for more ideas on how to treat them.

Nerve Pain Relief

> 4 drops lavender
> 3 drops marjoram
> 3 drops helichrysum (if available)
> 2 drops chamomile
> 1 ounces vegetable oil

Combine ingredients. Apply as needed for relief.

Arthritic Pain Formula

> 4 drops birch
> 3 drops marjoram
> 3 drops lavender
> 2 drops ginger
> 1 ounces vegetable oil

Combine ingredients. Apply as needed for relief.

PMS AND MENSTRUAL CRAMPS

Any woman who has experienced menstrual cramps or symptoms of pre-menstrual syndrome (PMS) knows how uncomfortable both conditions can be. Fortunately, there are essential oils that reduce painful cramping and most of the problems accompanying PMS. Research shows some oils lower prostaglandin 2, a hormonal substance that causes blood-sugar imbalances, headaches, bowel changes, nausea, breast tenderness and cysts, joint pain, and water retention, while contributing to moodiness, irritability, and alcohol cravings—all common PMS symptoms. Among the essential oils that help reduce menstrual cramps are muscle relaxants such as chamomile, lavender, marjoram, and melissa. The best way to use them? I suggest a long, relaxing bath or massage.

Essential Oils for Cramps and PMS

chamomile	garlic	marjoram
cinnamon	ginger	melissa
cloves	lavender	thyme

Menstrual Cramp and PMS Oil

> 12 drops lavender
> 6 drops marjoram
> 4 drops chamomile
> 4 drops ginger
> 2 ounces vegetable oil

Combine ingredients and apply as often as needed over cramping area. This formula is also excellent for the low-back pain that sometimes accompanies menstrual cramps.

SINUS AND RESPIRATORY CONGESTION

Ninety percent of respiratory ailments are caused by viruses. Fortunately, several essential oils inhibit viruses, including most of the viruses responsible for flus and colds. Some oils contribute to loosening and eliminating lung and sinus congestion, making them excellent cold, flu, and hay fever remedies. Along with essential oil of peppermint and eucalyptus, anise reduces coughing and also relaxes muscle spasms around the lungs.

Anyone who has ever sniffed black pepper, eucalyptus, peppermint, or pine knows how just smelling these essential oils helps clear the sinuses. Cypress will dry up a persistent runny nose. As an extra benefit, all these oils fight the bacterial infections that so often accompany a cold or flu.

A throat spray or gargle brings the essential oils into direct contact with a sore throat or laryngitis. Vapor balms, in addition to carrying the oils, increase circulation and warmth in the chest, important factors in fighting infection. Warm, moist steam opens nasal and bronchial passages, making it easier to breathe, and brings the essential oils to infected sinuses and lungs. Essential oils can be used in a humidifier, or on low heat in a pan of water, to disinfect the air. *CAUTION:* black pepper, cinnamon, and thyme are fine in a vapor balm or gargle, but steaming with them can irritate the respiratory tract.

When steaming is impractical, use a natural nasal inhaler. You can buy one in natural-food stores, or make your own with the formula below.

Antiviral Essential Oils

bergamot	cinnamon	hyssop
black pepper	eucalyptus	melissa

| peppermint | rosemary | thyme |
| ravensara | tea tree | |

Essential Oils for Congestion

anise	eucalyptus	pine
benzoin	frankincense	sandalwood
black pepper	myrrh	tea tree
cypress	peppermint	thyme

Steam

3–6 drops essential oils
3 cups water

Bring water to a simmer in a pan. Place a towel over the back of your head and tuck the ends around the pot so the steam is captured inside the improvised "tent." Take deep breaths of the steam for as long as is comfortable.

Homemade Nasal Inhaler

5 drops eucalyptus
1/4 teaspoon coarse salt

Place the salt in a small vial (glass is best) with a tight lid, and add oil. The salt will absorb the oil and provide a convenient way of carrying the oil without spilling it. When needed, open the vial and inhale deeply. This same technique can be used with any essential oil.

Throat Spray/Gargler

5 drops thyme or sage
1/2 cup water
1/2 teaspoon salt

Shake well to disperse the oils before gargling. Gargle a small amount throughout the day.

Vapor Rub

12 drops eucalyptus
5 drops peppermint
5 drops thyme
1 ounce olive oil

Combine ingredients in a glass bottle. Shake well to mix oils evenly. Gently massage into chest and throat.

VARICOSE VEINS AND HEMORRHOIDS

Medical doctors offer patients with varicose veins or hemorrhoids little hope of recovery except through surgery. I have seen essential oils of chamomile, palmarosa, myrtle, frankincense, and cypress (best when added to an infused oil of St. John's wort) reduce the size of blood vessels associated with these problems, and also ease the inflammation and pain they cause. If the skin is ulcerated and broken, apply a compress of carrot seed essential oil. With either condition, be sure to work on ways to improve your circulation with increased exercise, improved diet, and a good herbal program.

Varicose Vein and Hemorrhoid Formula

6 drops cypress
3 drops myrtle
3 drops German chamomile
2 drops frankincense (optional)
1 ounce St. John's wort herb oil (or vegetable oil)

Combine ingredients. Apply externally. You can buy St. John's wort infused oil in natural-food stores.

Carrot Seed Compress

8 drops carrot seed
1/2 cup water

Add essential oil to water. Slosh a soft cloth in water, wring out, fold, and place over ulcerated veins.

Mother and Baby Care

The gentlest oils are your best choices for use on babies and young children, and also during pregnancy. For pregnant women and children, use only one-third the amount of essential oils required in similar formulas for adults. Be cautious about using essential oils at all during the first trimester of pregnancy; even oils that are generally considered safe may be too stimulating for a woman who is prone to miscarriage.

Essential Oils for Mother and Child

chamomile	jasmine	sandalwood
citruses	lavender	spearmint
frankincense	neroli	ylang-ylang
geranium	rose	

PREGNANCY

Massage and aromatherapy can help prevent stretch marks from forming as a pregnant woman's belly expands. If possible, apply the belly oil at least twice per day. Lavender is one of the gentlest essential oils, and excellent for keeping skin supple. It is also an old companion in the birthing room, and many women still appreciate being massaged with this oil during labor to help them relax. After birth, add a couple drops of clary sage to the belly oil to help counter post-partum depression.

Belly Oil

1/2 ounce cocoa butter
4 ounces vegetable oil
25 drops (1/4 teaspoon) lavender
5 drops neroli
1600 IU vitamin E

Put oil and cocoa butter in a pan over low heat. Melt the cocoa butter (sold in drug stores), then remove from heat. Stir in essential oils and vitamin E, and bottle. (Obtain vitamin E by popping open a few capsules or buying it as a liquid.) Massage your belly with the oil—or get someone to do it for you—at least once per day.

DIAPER RASH

Aromatherapy baby oil and powder are good ways to protect your baby from diaper rash. The oil forms a barrier on the skin to repel moisture; the powder absorbs moisture and prevents chafing. Use one or the other with every diaper change, or more often if needed.

Baby oil also makes an excellent massage oil for babies. However, commercial baby oils and ointments are typically made from petroleum-based mineral oil, a good machinery lubricant but questionable for use on the skin. By the same token, commercial baby powders often contain talc, which may be contaminated with asbestos or other harmful substances. A good alternative is to make your own baby oils and powders.

Herbal Baby Oil

  12 drops lavender
  4 drops chamomile
  4 ounces vegetable oil
Combine ingredients.

Fragrant Baby Powder

  25 drops (1/4 teaspoon) lavender
  1/2 pound corn starch

Put the corn starch in a plastic zip-lock bag and drop in the essential oils. Tightly close the bag and toss back and forth to distribute the oil, breaking up any clumps by pressing them with your fingers through the bag. Let stand at least four days, continuing to break up the clumps. Spice or salt shakers with large perforations in the lid make good powder dispensers.

HIVES

Hives—rash-like skin bumps that can drive kids (as well as their parents) crazy with itching—are a symptom of food allergy. Of course, it is a good idea to address the dietary causes of the problem, but the immediate need is to stop the itching. Wash off the child's skin with the following herbal wash. If this does not provide enough relief, apply the herbal poultice. You may find that even a child who normally objects to having a poultice smeared on his or her skin will accept whatever will stop the itching of hives.

Hives Skin Wash

10 drops chamomile
3 tablespoons baking soda
2 cups elderflower tea

First make an extra strong tea by pouring 2-1/2 cups of boiling water over four teaspoons of elderflower. Steep 15 minutes, then strain out the herbs. Now add the baking soda and chamomile. Use a soft cloth or skin sponge to apply on irritated skin until itching is alleviated. If you don't have elderflower to make the tea, use another soothing herb such as calendula. If no herbs are available, add the chamomile to plain water. Lavender essential oil can be substituted for chamomile if necessary.

Hives Skin Poultice

3 tablespoons bentonite clay
1 tablespoon slippery-elm-bark powder
1/4 cup of the hives skin wash (above)

Stir all the ingredients into a paste and wait about five minutes for it to thicken. Apply to irritated skin with your fingers or a tongue depressor. Let dry on skin; leave at least 45 minutes before washing.

RESTLESSNESS

One of the most relaxing treatments for children before bedtime—or anytime—is a warm lavender and chamomile essential-oil bath. To completely relax the child, follow the bath with an aromatherapy massage. You can also send children off to dreamland with a "dilly pillow" filled with the herlbs lavender, hops, chamomile, and dill.

Relaxing Bath

2 drops lavender
1 drop orange
1 drop chamomile

Add oils directly to bath and stir to distribute.

Relaxing Children's Massage Oil

3 drops lavender
2 drops orange
1 drop chamomile
1 drop ylang-ylang (optional)
2 ounces vegetable oil

Combine ingredients. Use for massage as needed.

Dilly Pillow

equal parts:
lavender flowers
hops strobilus
chamomile flowers
dill seeds
5-by-10-inch piece of cloth.

Fold the cloth in half (so it measures 5-by-5 inches) and sew the edges, leaving a few inches open for stuffing. Combine the herbs and stuff them into the pillow, then sew closed. Slip this pillow inside the child's pillowcase. Add thyme to prevent nightmares.

TEETHING

To relieve teething pain, rub the child's gums with a little clove-bud essential oil on your finger. This can be hot stuff, so make sure the oil is diluted enough by trying it in your own mouth first.

Teething Oil

1 drop orange
4 drops clove bud
1 tablespoon vegetable oil

Combine ingredients. Rub a few drops on painful gums. Repeat every half hour or so. If your child refuses the clove teething oil, try replacing the clove with chamomile, which is a less effective pain reliever but isn't hot like the clove.

Home Improvements

Aromatherapy has long been used to keep houses smelling fresh. It can also be used as a natural repellent to keep away pesky insects such as mosquitoes and moths. Not only is it easy to make your own potpourris, room fresheners, and bug repellents, the ones you make with real essential oils smell much better than the synthetics that are commonly used in commercial products.

AIR FRESHENERS

Modern potpourris owe most of their fragrance to essential oils added to dried herbs. They make attractive room fresheners when set around the house. You can also place essential oils on a light bulb (or purchase light-bulb rings, which make the scent last longer), in diffuser, or into a simmering potpourri cooker.

If you want a stronger freshener, use an aromatherapy spray instead. One of the formulas below is a room disinfectant that can be sprayed in a sick room or used on a kitchen counter. You may also change the recommended essential oils to achieve a desired fragrance, or choose an oil that impacts the emotions. (I know one mom who sprays the kids' bedrooms every evening with a soothing chamomile and ylang-ylang mix.)

The first formula is a basic recipe for potpourri. Orris root, which helps preserve the fragrance, has a light, violet-like scent that blends with almost any fragrance, yet is not overpowering. An essential oil of orris is produced, but it is quite rare and costly, so I use the root instead.

Potpourri

1 cup dried plant material
1 tablespoon orris root
1/4 teaspoon essential oil

Use any combination of attractive flowers, leaves, or cones for the dried plant material. Add orris root and essential oils. Keep in a closed container for several days, enough time for the scent to permeate the plant material. This potpourri should stay fragrant for many months. When it gets faint, revive it with a few more drops of essential oil. For a simmering potpourri, double the quantity of essential oil, using 1/2 teaspoon per cup. Note: Some people complain about being allergic to orris. There are several essential oil fixatives suitable for potpourri, including patchouli, sandalwood, benzoin, clary sage, balsam of Peru, balsam of tolu, vetiver, and vetiver.

Disinfectant Room Spray

4 drops eucalyptus (or tea tree)
3 drops lavender
2 drops bergamot
2 drops thyme
1 drop peppermint
2 ounces water

Add essential oils to water and keep in a spritzer bottle (sold in most drug stores and in some cosmetics stores). Shake well a few times per day for several days after making the spray, and right before each use. Some of the oil will still float on the top, but because the tube in the spritzer bottle extends to the bottom of the bottle, this should not present a problem.

BUG REPELLENTS

I won't claim that aromatherapy bug repellents work better than standard drug-store varieties, but they are a good alternative to rubbing toxic chemical repellents into your skin. Mosquitoes, ticks, and many other insect pests hate the smell of especially pungent essential oils such as citronella; unfortunately, so do quite a few people. I find that these pungent smells turn more fragrant with the addition of geranium, which itself is a bug repellent.

Another way to reduce the insect population is a citronella candle. Impregnated with citronella, these candles release the scent as they burn. They are available from most camping and household stores and catalogs, or you can make your own (see below).

Natural Mosquito Repellents

cedarwood	eucalyptus	pennyroyal
citronella	geranium	

Bug Repellent

1/4 teaspoon citronella
1/4 teaspoon eucalyptus
1/8 teaspoon pennyroyal
1/8 teaspoon cedar
1/8 teaspoon geranium
2 ounces carrier oil

Combine ingredients. Since this repellent will sting eyes, mouth, and other sensitive tissues, be sure to keep the oil away from them (e.g., don't rub your eyes right after applying the formula with your fingers). This repellent will last for at least a year.

Citronella Candle

votive candle
20 drops citronella

Using a glass dropper, drip the oil on the candle's wick. Give the wick twenty-four hours to absorb the oil, and the candle is ready to burn.

MOTH REPELLENT

The traditional way to keep moths out of your woolens is to store them in a cedarwood chest during the summer. The wood of camphor has a similar repellent effect on clothes moths; camphor chests have long been used in China to protect woolens and silk. In India, patchouli keeps moths out of Oriental carpets—in fact, when Europeans started producing cheaper imitations of these rugs, wary buyers knew they weren't authentic because they didn't smell like patchouli.

Modern moth balls are harsh, displeasing imitations of camphor. The problem is that they not only make your clothes and blankets smell terrible, but are quite toxic. It is far better to use a pleasant-smelling, natural alternative.

Natural Moth Repellents

camphor	patchouli	tansy
cedarwood	sage	wormwood
lavender	southernwood	

Wool-Moth Repellent

20 drops cedarwood
8 drops lavender
8 drops patchouli or sage
1 dozen cotton balls

Combine essential oils and place about three drops on each cotton ball. Store in a closed container for a couple of days. Place with clothes, about six for an average-size box or suitcase. For more attractive moth balls, tie a small fabric square around each cotton ball.

FLEA CONTROL

The first time I used aromatherapy flea control on my dog Freckles, I expected to see fleas jumping everywhere. They didn't, and when I examined his fur, I saw they were all dead. You may need to repeat the shampoo in a few days, since this treatment kills fleas but not all the eggs. *IMPORTANT:* If you have a flea infestation, vacuum anywhere the pet spends time, then spray the area with a cedarwood repellent.

Go easy putting products containing essential oils directly on your pet's fur—especially cats, since they lick their coats so much. And never put them directly on an animal's skin. It is far better to put a few drops of flea-repelling essential oils on a collar (see below) than directly on the animal.

One bonus to discouraging fleas is that you will be keeping ticks away at the same time.

NATURAL FLEA REPELLENTS

bay	citronella	lemon
camphor	eucalyptus	pennyroyal
cedarwood		

Flea Bath

1/2 cup unfragranced pet shampoo
1/2 teaspoon orange

Combine ingredients. Lather your pet well, because the shampoo acts as a carrier for the essential oil, and the suds help to trap the fleas. Fleas have a tendency to migrate toward the head, so be sure to carefully shampoo the face and especially the neck. You can also use people shampoo for this recipe.

Cedarwood Spray

1 cup water
20 drops cedarwood

Mix together and, because essential oils and water do not mix easily, shake well before each spray.

Flea Collar

10 drops pennyroyal
5 drops citronella
5 drops eucalyptus
5 drops cedarwood
Soft, absorbent cotton rope

Combine essential oils. With a dropper, run a thin bead of essential oils along a leash or a segment of rope that is long enough to comfortably go around your animal's neck. (Make sure that it isn't so loose that the animal could get it caught on elome datacompsomething.) Let dry about 30 minutes and tie on. The repellent effects will last a week or two.

Flea Powder

20 drops cedarwood
1 cup cornstarch

Add essential oil to cornstarch and stir to distribute. Let sit a few days, enough time for the oils to dissipate through the cornstarch. Rub into the animal's fur. You could use some of the other repellent essential oils for this formula, but I choose cedar because it is less toxic should the animal decide to lick its fur.

Materia Medica
SIXTY COMMON ESSENTIAL OILS

ANGELICA (*Angelica archangelica*)
Magical powers have been attributed to this "root of the Holy Ghost," once a common flavoring and apothecary drug. The oil distilled from the seed of this herb is spicy and peppery. The root oil, which is stronger and slightly more expensive than the seed, smells earthier and more herbal. The fragrance of angelica gives depressed people a new outlook on life. Both seed and root oils regulate menstruation and digestion, and also stop coughing. However, use angelica very carefully because it can overstimulate the nervous system. The root oil also contains the photosensitive agent bergapten.

ANISE (*Pimpinella anisum*)
The delightful licorice-like scent and taste of this herb flavors pharmaceuticals, confections, toothpaste, "licorice" candy (in the U.S.), and alcoholic beverages such as French anisette and Greek ouzo. Anise reduces muscle spasms, indigestion, and coughing. It is also mildly estrogenic, and an aphrodisiac. It increases breast milk, balances emotions, induces sleep, and helps overcome nervousness and workaholic stress. Anise is even said to improve your sense of humor and overcome heartache. Large quantities, however, may be narcotic, slow down circulation, and cause skin rashes in sensitive people.

BASIL (*Ocimum basilicum*)
Distilled from the leaves and flowering tops, this familiar sweet-and-spicy kitchen herb relieves headaches, sinus congestion, temporary loss of smell, nausea (even from

chemotherapy), indigestion, sore muscles, and the herpes and shingles viruses. Basil gently stimulates adrenal glands, menstruation, childbirth, and production of breast milk. Basil reduces stress, rattled nerves, hysteria, and mental, fatigue while increasing confidence, decisiveness, positive thoughts, and awareness of one's surrounding. Large doses can be over-stimulating and may stupefy.

BAY *(Laurus nobilis)*

A pungent, spicy aroma is distilled from the leaf and, occasionally, the berry of the bay tree (also called bay laurel), which stimulants lymph and circulation while relieving sinus and lung congestion. It improves the memory; hence, the Ancient Greeks placed bay wreaths on the heads of scholars—and headache sufferers! The priestesses at Delphi sat over burning bay fumes to induce prophetic visions. If you purchase "bay," it is most likely bay rum *(Pimenta racemosa)*, which is cooler and sweeter and is used to scent colognes, soaps, and cosmetics. Unlike true bay, bay rum can irritate delicate skin and mucous membranes.

BENZOIN *(Styrax benzoin)*

The sweet, vanilla-like absolute is solvent-extracted from the tree's gum resin. In India, benzoin is sacred to the Brahma-Shiva-Vishnu triad of deities. Malays use it to fend off evil during rice-harvesting ceremonies. It is antiseptic and anti-fungal, protects chapped skin, and increases skin elasticity. It is helpful for those who feel anxious, emotionally blocked, lonely, or exhausted, especially after a life crisis. Balsam of tolu *(Myroxylon balsamum)* and balsam of Peru *(M. balsamum,* var. *Pereirae)* are gum resins with similar aromas and properties. Avoid benzoin oils thinned with ethyl glycol.

BERGAMOT (*Citrus bergamia*)

This fresh, clean scent is cold-pressed from the almost-ripe rind of a small, green citrus fruit. Named after Bergamo, Italy, where the oil originated, it scents colognes, and flavors Earl Grey tea and some candies. It is also used as a deodorizer. Bergamot aids digestion, and reduces inflammation and infection in the genito-urinary system, mouth, throat, and skin. It kills several viruses, including those responsible for flu, herpes, shingles, and chickenpox, and is a traditional Italian folk medicine to treat fever and intestinal worms. It counters depression, anxiety, insomnia, and compulsive behavior cycles, including eating disorders. Bergamot contains photosensitizing bergapten, although a bergapten-free essential oil is available. Don't confuse *Citrus bergamia* with common garden bergamot (*Monarda didyma*), also known as "bee balm."

BIRCH (*Betula lenta*)

The bark of this tree is the source of commercial "wintergreen" oil, since the chemistry, properties, and fragrance of both oils is the same. Birch relieves muscular and arthritic pain, softens skin, soothes irritation and psoriasis, and eliminates dandruff. While people tend to associate birch's scent with medicine or candy, it can be toxic in large amounts, so use carefully.

CAMPHOR (*C. camphora*)

Unlike harsh, synthetic moth balls, the leaves and bark of this tree produce a pleasant oil, woodsy with a hint of cardamom. Camphor counters shock and depression, and helps to focus your attention. Arab cultures use it to reduce sexual desire. White camphor is a heart stimulant and potentially toxic, so use it cautiously—and *don't* use the even more toxic brown or yellow camphor produced from heavier parts of the oil.

CARROT SEED *(Daucus carota)*

A fruity, sharp, pungent fragrance distilled from the seeds of Queen Anne's lace, ancestor of the common carrot, carrot seed stimulates circulation and treats some genito-urinary and digestive disorders. It is also gaining popularity for its ability to enhance skin tone and elasticity, and decrease dryness, wrinkles, dermatitis, eczema, rashes, and even certain pre-cancerous skin conditions.

CEDARWOOD *(Cedrus species)*

This soft, woodsy fragrance scents soap and cologne, serving as an astringent for oily skin, acne, dandruff, dermatitis, bites, and itching. Cedar also helps in cases of respiratory and urinary infections. Emotionally, it increases self-respect, integrity, stability, meditation, and intuition, while relieving stress, aggression, and dependency. It repels wool moths and other insects. Moroccan cedar *(C. lbani)* is the legendary "cedar of Lebanon" prized by ancient cultures. The pine-like Atlantic cedar *(C. atlantica)* is from Morocco. Himalayan cedarwood *(C. deodara)* is warm and spicy, and the least toxic cedar oil. Juniper *(Juniperus virginiana)* is actually the source of most commercial "cedar" oil—and of wood pencils. *CAUTION:* Avoid all cedars during pregnancy.

CHAMOMILE, GERMAN
(Matricaria recutita, formerly M. chamomilla)

A sweet, herbaceous, and apple-like aroma is distilled from chamomile's flowers. Chamomile reduces inflammation due to sensitive skin; rashes; boils; sore muscles, tendons, and joints; headaches; asthma; allergies; hemorrhoids; and enlarged veins. It also treats indigestion, light constipation, PMS, menstrual pain, ulcers, and liver damage. A strong antidepressant, chamomile helps overcome over-sensitivity, stress, anxiety, hysteria, insomnia, suppressed anger, and hyperactivity. The more expensive German chamomile oil is blue, while the closely related Roman chamomile (*Chamaemelum nobile*, formerly *Anthemis nobilis*) is pale yellow. Also sold as "blue chamomile" are *Ormenis multicaulis*, *Tanacetum anuum*, and *Artemisia arborescens*). The last two are potentially toxic, so use them very carefully.

CINNAMON (*Cinnamomum zeylanicum*)

Distilled from the tree's leaf or bark, cinnamon is a sweet, spicy-hot fragrance. The bark is hotter-smelling, hotter-tasting (it can irritate skin and especially mucous membranes), and more expensive. Cinnamon stops menstrual cramps, diarrhea, and genito-urinary infections, while increasing sweating and providing heat for liniments. It is an aphrodisiac that relieves tension, steadies nerves, and invigorates the senses. Small amounts spice up Oriental perfume blends. Cassia, or *kuei pi* (*C. cassia*), is an inexpensive substitute from China used in medicine, seasoning, incense, and cola drinks

CITRONELLA (*Citronella nardus*)

The sharp lemon scent of this grass-like herb is used extensively in cleaning products because it is less expensive than true lemon. It treats colds, infections, and oily complexions, and is considered a physical and emotional purifier. The most popular use of citronella is to ward off insects, especially mosquitoes. It often adulterates expensive lemon verbena and melissa, although it is much harsher and more camphoric, and can irritate the skin.

CLARY SAGE *(Salvia sclarea)*

Although clary is related to common sage, it is quite different: relaxing and euphoric, enhancing dreams and producing smiles. Distilled from the herb's flowering tops, clary's wine-like scent is sweet and heady. Clary eases muscle and nervous tension, pain, menstrual cramps, PMS, and menopause problems such as hot flashes, while slightly stimulating the adrenal glands. It also has estrogenic action. In Europe, it is used as a sore throat remedy. Clary helps rejuvenate hair and mature or inflamed skin, and reduces dandruff. It helps in cases of panic, paranoia, mental fatigue, general debility, post-partum depression, and PMS. Avoid large amounts, which can stupefy, and don't combine clary with alcohol.

CLOVE BUD
(Syzygium aromaticum, formerly *Eugenia caryophyllata)*

The spicy, hot scent is distilled from the immature buds, leaves, or stems of the tree. Europeans, East Indians, and Chinese still use clove bud oil to sweeten their breath and eliminate toothache. It also treats flu, sore muscles, arthritis, colds, and bronchial congestion, and is a heating liniment. The eugenol from clove is made into drugs that kill germs and pain. As a stimulant, clove helps overcome nervousness, stress, mental fatigue, and poor memory. Avoid the leaf, which can irritate skin and mucous membranes.

CORIANDER *(Coriandrum sativum)*

The seed of this culinary herb yields a spicy, sharp, distinct fragrance. It soothes inflammation, rheumatic pain, headaches, cystitis, flu, and diarrhea, and is generally antiseptic. Although it was used as a love potion in Medieval times, the fourteenth-century nuns of St. Just included coriander in "Carmelite water," a combined cologne and facial toner. It still scents soaps and deodorants. Uplifting and motivating, the scent of coriander also relieves stress.

CYPRESS (*Cupressus sempervirens*)

Distilled from the needles, twigs or cones of the tree, the odor is sharp, pungent, pine-like, and spicy. Cypress is found in men's cologne and aftershave. The smoke was inhaled in southern Europe to relieve sinus congestion, while the Chinese chewed the small cones to reduce gum inflammation. Cypress helps circulation problems such as low blood pressure, varicose veins, and hemorrhoids. It alleviates laryngitis, spasmodic coughing, lung congestion, excessive menstruation, urinary problems, and cellulite. Used as a deodorant, cypress reduces excessive sweating. It also eases insomnia and grief, and increases emotional stamina, helping one to move on after an emotional crisis.

DILL (*Anethum graveolens*)

A sharp herbal scent is distilled from the seed of this culinary herb to treat obesity, water retention, and indigestion. Early Americans chewed the seeds to inhibit their appetite during long church services. Babies with colic were once given "gripe water"—a syrup of dill, fennel, and baking soda—and laid to sleep on fragrant "dilly pillows" of dill, lavender, and chamomile (see page 67). Dill also refines the complexion.

EUCALYPTUS (*Eucalyptus globulus*)

Distilled from leaves and twigs, this essential oil is pungent, sharp, and somewhat camphoric. Eucalyptus oil (or its component eucalyptol) goes into industrial preparations, aftershaves, colognes, mouthwashes, liniments, and vapor rubs. It treats sinus and throat infection, fever, flu, chickenpox, and herpes. It is excellent on oily complexion, especially acne, boils, and insect bites, and for killing lice. The scent alone increases energy, countering physical debility and emotional imbalance.

FENNEL (*Foeniculum vulgare*)

Distilled from the herb's seeds, the scent is herbaceous, sweet, and licorice-like. Fennel decreases obesity, water retention, urinary-tract problems, indigestion, and colic. Its hormonal properties (mostly estrogenic) increase mother's milk and slightly stimulate the adrenal glands. It refines the mature complexion and heals bruises. Stimulating and revitalizing, fennel increases self-motivation and enlivens the personality. Because large amounts can over-excite the nervous system and even cause convulsions, use fennel carefully—and not at all if you have nervous-system problems or epilepsy.

FIR (*Abies alba*)

The oil can be distilled from the twigs or needles of several different fir trees, as well as from spruces, pines, and other conifers. Fir soothes muscle and rheumatism pain, increases poor circulation, inhibits bronchial, genito-urinary, and skin infections, and lessens asthma and coughing. It enhances the senses both of being grounded and of being elevated, increases intuition, and releases energy and emotional blocks.

FRANKINCENSE (*Boswellia carteri*)

This small tree grows on the rocky hillsides of Yemen, Oman, and Somalia. When distilled, the oleo gum resin produces a soft, basalmic oil. Frankincense treats lung and genito-urinary complaints, ulcers, chronic diarrhea, breast cysts, and excessive menstruation. Use it on mature skin, acne, fungal infections, boils, hard-to-heal wounds, and scars. For centuries, frankincense has been used to increase spirituality, mental perception, meditation, prayer, and consciousness. It fortifies and soothes the spirit, slows and deepens breathing, and is relaxing. It is said to release past links and subconscious stress.

GERANIUM *(Pelargonium graveoloens)*

The oil is distilled from the leaves of this herb (known as "rose geranium") and smells like a combination of rose, citrus, and herb. A light adrenal-gland stimulant and hormonal normalizer, geranium treats PMS, menopause, fluid retention, breast engorgement, and sterility, and helps to regulate blood pressure. A versatile skin treatment, it reduces inflammation, infection, eczema, acne, burn injuries, bleeding, scarring, stretch marks, shingles, herpes, and ringworm. It is also said to delay wrinkling. Geranium relieves anxiety, depression, discontent, irrational behavior, and stress. It is also used to heal a passive-aggressive nature and to enhances one's perception of time and space. Some aromatherapists describe it as sedative, while others consider it stimulating, but it probably is a balancer.

GINGER *(Zingiber officinale)*

Distilled from the rhizome, the fragrance is spicy, warm, and sharp. Ginger treats colds, fevers, appetite loss, nausea, inflammation, and genito-urinary and lung infections. Studies show that ginger increases the absorption of herbs in the body, and helps to protect the liver. It is a stimulant and an aphrodisiac, and is used in warming liniments.

GRAPEFRUIT *(C. paradisi)*

The oil that is pressed from the peel of this fruit encourages weight loss and gall bladder activity. Grapefruit is a favorite with children, and very useful for anyone undergoing inner-child psychological work.

HELICHRYSUM *(Helichrysum angustifolium)*

A pleasant spicy, sweet, almost fruity fragrance is distilled from the flowers of this everlasting, sometimes called "immortelle." It treats the infection and inflammation of chronic cough, bronchitis, fever, muscle pain, arthritis, phlebitis, and liver problems, as well as countering allergic reactions such as asthma. Use helichrysum on acne, on scar tissue, on bruises, on couperose or mature skin, and on burns to stimulate production of new cells. The scent lifts one from depression, lethargy, and nervous exhaustion, and helps alleviate stress. Some aromatherapists say it helps detoxify from drugs, including nicotine. The French oil is green, while the less-refined Yugoslavian oil has an orange hue.

INULA, SWEET *(Inula graveolens or I. odorata)*

Distilled from the plant's root, the oil is a rich blue-green with a pungent odor that faintly resembles eucalyptus. Inula relieves muscle tension, inflammation, sinus congestion, bronchitis, and high blood pressure. A compound derived from inula is used in Europe to treat intestinal worms. It also relieves skin rashes, herpes, and itching. An essential oil is produced from the closely related medicinal herb elecampane *(Inula helenium)*, but tends to cause skin reactions.

JASMINE *(Jasminum officinalis and J. grandiflorum)*

An enfleurage, an absolute, and a concrete are made from the plant's blossoms, whose complex fragrance is fruity, floral, and sweetly exotic, and is found in many expensive perfumes. The synthetic version is so harsh it demands a touch of the true oil to soften it. Jasmine is a nervous-system sedative that reduces menstrual cramps and is sometimes used to treat prostate problems. Good for sensitive and mature complexions, jasmine also soothes headaches, insomnia, and depression, dissolving apathy, indifference, and lack of confidence by increasing the sense of self-worth. Jasmine is an aphrodisiac and also increases receptivity. The most prized oil comes from France and Italy, although about 80 percent is Egyptian.

JUNIPER (*Juniperus communis*)

The berries of this North American shrub offer the highest-quality oil, although needles and branches are sometimes used. Its pungent, herbaceous, peppery odor is pine-like and camphoric. Juniper treats arteriosclerosis, rheumatic pain, general debility, varicose veins, hemorrhoids, fluid retention, cellulite, and genito-urinary tract and bronchial infections. It is suitable for treatment of acne, eczema, and greasy hair or dandruff. Juniper provides a feeling of protection when the demands of others pull too strongly, and is suggested for those who experience mental or emotional fatigue, insomnia, or anxiety. It can overstimulate the kidneys, so choose a less toxic oil when kidneys are inflamed.

LABDANUM (*Cistus ladanifer*)

This is the "rock rose" grown in North American gardens. The leaves and twigs are boiled, and the resin skimmed off and aged, to produce a resinoid with a warm, spicy, balsamic odor, sometimes used as a fixative in perfumes. Oil distilled from the leaves is called "cistus", a nervous-system sedative used to treat rheumatism, colds, coughs, menstrual problems, inflamed kidneys, and hemorrhoids. Labdanum is also antiseptic on wounds, acne, dermatitis, and boils. It is both emotionally elevating and grounding, improving meditation and intuition, and raising consciousness. It calms the nerves, promotes sleep, and is an aphrodisiac. Don't confuse labdanum with *laudanum*, or tincture of opium poppy.

LAVENDER *(Lavandula angustifolia)*

Distilled from the herb's flower buds, this sweetly floral aroma is also herbal, with balsamic undertones. Lavender treats lung, sinus, and vaginal infections (including candida), and relieves muscle pain, headaches, insect bites, cystitis, and other types of inflammation. It is also used for digestive disturbances, including colic, and boosts immunity. A skin-cell regenerator, lavender prevents scarring and stretch marks, and has a reputation for slowing wrinkles. It is suitable for all complexion types, as well as for burns, sun damage, wounds, rashes, and skin infections. Specific for central-nervous-system problems, lavender has been used to help nervousness, exhaustion, insomnia, irritability, depression, and even manic depression.

LEMON *(Citrus limonum)*

This distinctive oil, cold-pressed from the fresh peel, is antioxidant, preservative, and antiseptic, countering both viral and bacterial infections. Lemon treats hypertension and increases the rate of metabolism, relieving congested lymph, excessive stomach activity, water retention, and weight gain, and increasing mineral absorption and immunity. Lemon helps oily complexions, bruises, and skin impurities and infections. Like other citruses, it is antidepressive, increasing general well-being and the sense of humor. It also dissipates feelings of impurity or indecisiveness, and can stimulate emotional purging. The only caution is that it can be photosensitizing to some skins.

LEMONGRASS *(Cymbopogon citratus)*

Distilled from partly dried herb, lemongrass oil has a slightly bitter fragrance that is used in cosmetics, deodorants, and soaps (including Ivory). Lemongrass is antiseptic and treats pain resulting from indigestion, rheumatism, nervous-system conditions, and headaches. It counters oily hair, acne, skin infections, scabies, and ringworm. The fragrance is sedating and soothing. Lemongrass is non-toxic, but produces skin sensitivity in some people.

LIME *(C. aurantifolia)*

The fragrance of this citrus fruit is similar to lemon, but smoother. Lime is motivating, relieving depression and increasing morale. Unlike other citruses, the peel may be distilled or pressed. Lime is slightly photosensitizing to some skins.

MARJORAM

(Origanum marjorana, formerly *Marjorana hortensis)*

Distilled from leaves of the culinary herb, the aroma is sweet-but-herbal and sharp, hinting of camphor. A sedative, marjoram eases muscle spasms, including tics and menstrual cramps, and relieves headaches (especially migraines), stiff joints, spasmodic coughs, and high blood pressure. It also counters colds, flu, and laryngitis, and is slightly laxative. Use it on the skin to tend bruises, burns, inflammation, and fungal and bacterial infections. Marjoram helps those who feel emotionally unstable, prone to hysteria, physically debilitated, or irritable—especially due to outside stimuli. Use it to ease loneliness, rejection, or a broken heart. (Old texts say that overuse may even deaden the emotions.) Note: Sometimes the much harsher oregano is commercially sold as marjoram.

MELISSA *(Melissa officinalis)*

Distilled from leaves of the herb lemon balm, melissa's sweet smell is soft and lemony. Not easily distilled, this expensive oil is often adulterated with lemon or citronella. It was the main ingredient in the famous "Carmelite water," a facial toner made by nuns in the Middle Ages. Melissa treats indigestion, lung congestion, high blood pressure, menstrual problems, and infertility. It fights inflammation, and viral infections such as strep, herpes, and chickenpox. Shock, distress, depression, nervousness, and insomnia are helped by its sedative properties.

MYRRH *(Commiphora myrrha)*

The tree gum is distilled into a warm, spicy, deep, and slightly bitter-sweet oil. It helps with coughs, digestion, diarrhea, an overactive thyroid, scanty menstruation, and immunity. Externally, it treats wounds, gum disease, candida, chapped, cracked, or aged skin, eczema, bruises, skin infections, varicose veins, and ringworm. Myrrh has been used since antiquity to inspire prayer and meditation, and to fortify and revitalize the spirit.

MYRTLE *(Myrtus communis)*

Distilled from leaves, twigs and sometimes flowers, the spicy scent is slightly camphoric. Myrtle was the main ingredient in the sixteenth-century complexion treatment called "angel's water." It treats lung and respiratory infections, muscle spasms, and hemorrhoids. Myrtle is a treatment for oily complexions, acne, and varicose veins. The scent balances energy.

NEROLI (ORANGE BLOSSOM) *(Citrus aurantium)*

This sweet, spicy, and intensely heady fragrance is distilled from the blossoms of the bitter orange tree. It treats diarrhea, and circulation problems such as hemorrhoids and high blood pressure. It is used on mature and couperose skin to regenerate cells. One of the best aromatic anti-depressives, neroli counters emotional shock, mental confusion, nervous strain, anxiety, fear, and lack of confidence. It redirects one's energy in a positive direction, relieving fatigue and insomnia, and helps those who get upset without apparent reason. It is also used as an aphrodisiac. The bitter-orange essential oil produced from the fruit rind of the same tree is potentially photosensitizing to the skin.

ORANGE (Citrus sinensis)
Cold-pressed from the sweet orange peel, the familiar scent is perky and lively. Orange treats flu, colds, congested lymph, irregular heartbeat, and high blood pressure. The sedative fragrance counters depression, hysteria, shock, and nervous tension. Orange is good for oily complexions, although the oil can be slightly photosensitizing. An inferior oil comes from peel that has been pressed to make orange juice.

PALMAROSA (Cymbopogon martini)
The lemon-rose fragrance of this grass is reminiscent of the richer and more expensive rose geranium, which it is often used to adulterate. The scent varies greatly depending on its source. A cell regenerator, palmarosa balances oil production by any complexion type, but especially with acne or otherwise infected skin. Palmarosa treats stress and nervous exhaustion.

PATCHOULI (Pogostemon cablin)
Distilled from aged, fermented leaves, the aroma is heavy, earthy, woody, and musty. Patchouli reduces appetite, water

retention, and exhaustion. A cell rejuvenator and antiseptic, it treats acne, eczema, athlete's foot, inflamed, cracked or mature skin, inflammation, and dandruff. Patchouli counters nervousness and depression by putting problems into perspective and releasing pent-up emotions. It is also an aphrodisiac.

PETITGRAIN (*C. aurantium*)

Now distilled from the fragrant leaves and stems of the bitter orange, this oil originally came from the small, unripe fruit, hence the name (which means "little fruit"). Petitgrain resembles neroli, but is harsher, sharper, and less expensive. An antidepressant, petitgrain also increases perception and awareness, and re-establishes trust and self-confidence.

PEPPER, BLACK (*Piper nigrum*)

The oil is distilled from the same partly dried, unripe fruit we sprinkle on food. The scent is spicy, sharp, and slightly herbaceous. (A more fruity oil is produced from the fresh green fruit.) Pepper treats food poisoning, indigestion, colds, flu, urinary-tract infections, congested lungs, fevers, and poor circulation. It makes a warming liniment. The fragrance is emotionally stimulating and, some say, aphrodisiac. Though non-toxic, pepper can irritate the skin.

PEPPERMINT (*Mentha piperita*)

Distilled from leaves of the herb, the aroma is powerful, minty, peppery, and fresh. Peppermint relieves muscle spasms, inflammation, indigestion, nausea, irritable-bowel syndrome, and sinus and lung congestion. It also destroys bacteria, viruses, and parasites in the digestive tract. Small amounts stimulate the skin's oil production and relieve itching from ringworm, herpes, scabies, and poison oak and ivy. Peppermint is used in liniments, although too much can burn the skin. As a stimulant, the scent counters insomnia, shock, mental fogginess, lack of focus, and "stuck" emotions.

PINE *(Pinus species)*

The sharp fragrance from pine needles is produced from several species, but Scotch pine *(P. sylvestis)* is most popular for cleansing solutions, European bath preparations (it improves poor circulation), and liniments. Pine replaces apathy and anxiety with peacefulness and invigoration. It is sometimes used to reverse male impotence.

RAVENSARE *(Ravensara aromatica)*

Distilled from the leaves—and sometimes the fruit or bark—of this Madagascar spice tree, the scent is similar to eucalyptus, but more refined and less sharp. Ravensare is an antiseptic treatment for flu, bronchitis, viral infections (including shingles), viral hepatitis, sinus congestion, and acne. It also relieves muscle fatigue.

ROSE *(Rosa damascena, R. gallica, and other spices)*

This costly oil is distilled, or solvent extracted, from the blossoms. It treats asthma, hay fever, liver problems, nausea, most female disorders, and impotence. A cell rejuvenator, rose soothes and heals all complexion types, and has a reputation for slowing down the skin's aging. It is also strongly antiseptic and fights infection. Rose helps alleviate depression and lack of confidence, and is useful for treating relationship conflicts, envy, and intolerance. It is comforting, supportive during a crisis, and an aphrodisiac.

ROSEMARY *(Rosmarinus officinalis)*

This herb's aroma, distilled from the flowering tops or leaves, is herbal, sharp, and camphoric. Possibly the first cologne, it was the main ingredient in the famous cologne

"Hungary water," which doubled as a facial toner for dry or mature complexions. Rosemary gently stimulates poor circulation, low blood pressure and energy, the nervous system, the adrenal glands, and the gall bladder. It lowers cholesterol and relieves lung congestion, sore throat, and canker sores. It is used for sore muscles, rheumatism, cellulite, and parasites. Rosemary improves memory, confidence, perception, and creativity, and balances both mind and body. It prevents dizziness, dark thoughts, and nightmares, and helps in the recall of dreams. The smoke was once inhaled to counteract "brain weakness" and to stimulate spiritual awareness. There are several chemotypes with different properties.

ROSEWOOD *(Aniba rosaeodora)*
The pleasant fragrance distilled from this tropical tree's wood is sweet, woodsy, and rosy. Rosewood eases headaches, cold, fever, infections, vaginitis, and nausea. It rejuvenates cells and benefits all types of complexions. As an antidepressive, it encourages constructive emotional work and tranquillity. Rosewood is a rainforest tree, and there is therefore concern lest it be over-harvested.

SAGE *(Salvia officinalis)*
Distilled from the leaves of the kitchen herb, the odor is spicy, sharp, and herbal. Sage is an antiseptic that treats throat and mouth infections. Hormonal properties help regulate both the menstrual cycle and menopause symptoms, and decrease lactation. Sage was a Medieval nervous-system tonic for tics and epilepsy. In Ancient Crete, the burning leaves were inhaled to relieve asthma. It reduces perspiration, oily skin, and acne, and is reputed to encourage hair growth. Sage helps those suffering from

nervous debility, excessive sexual desire, grief, physical overexertion, and insomnia. It encourages inward focus. Sage contains the potentially neurotoxic thujone, so use it carefully and not on anyone prone to seizures.

SANDALWOOD (Santalum album)

Distilled from the tree's heartwood or roots, the scent is balsamic, soft, warm, and woody. Once a gonorrhea treatment, sandalwood is still used for genito-urinary infections. It counters inflammation, hemorrhoids, persistent coughs, nausea, throat problems, and some nerve pain. Suitable for all complexion types, sandalwood is useful on rashes, inflammation, acne, and chapped skin. It also treats depression, anxiety, and insomnia, and helps instill peaceful relaxation, openness, and a sense of "grounding."

SPEARMINT (M. spicata)

The spearmint aroma is less peppery and sharper than the closely-related peppermint. It is also slightly weaker in action, though it too is used as a stimulant. Spearmint brings back childhood joy and pleasant memories.

TANGERINE (C. reticulata)

Distilled peel of tangerine produces this lively citrus scent, which counters insomnia and digestive problems, and is especially safe for children and pregnant women. The leaves are also steam-distilled for "petitgrain mandarin." The closely related mandarin orange—whose scent is very similar, but slightly richer and fuller—comes from the same species.

TEA TREE (Melaleuca alternifolia)

The oil distilled from the leaves of this tree is similar to the closely related eucalyptus. A good immune tonic and a strong antiseptic, tea tree fights lung, genito-urinary, vaginal, sinus, mouth, and fungal infections, as well as viral infections such as herpes, shingles, chickenpox, candida, thrush, and influenza. Tea tree also treats diaper rash, acne, wounds, and insect bites, and protects the skin from radiation burns caused by cancer therapy. It is touted as one of the most non-irritating oils, but this varies with the species and the individual. It builds emotional strength, especially before an operation or during post-operative shock. "MQV" (*M. quinquenervia viridiflora*), which has a distinctively sweeter fragrance, is considered a stronger antiviral.

THUJA (*Thuja occidentalis*)
Known also as "cedar leaf" or "arbor vitae," the oil is distilled from the leaves, twigs, or bark of this small tree, or sometimes from a cultivar or closely related species. The fragrance falls somewhere between the softness of cedar and the sharpness of pine. Thuja eliminates warts and treats pelvic congestion, urinary infections, and enlarged prostate. Thuja contains a skin irritant that is potentially very toxic, so use it carefully—and not at all if you are prone to seizures.

THYME (*Thymus vulgaris*)
The scent, produced by distillation, is herbal, warm, almost sweet. Thyme is a strong anti-bacterial for mouth and lung infections, and destroys intestinal hookworms and roundworms. It relieves indigestion, coughs, and lung congestion, and was once a specific treatment for whooping cough. It is also a heating liniment. Thyme relieves mental instability, melancholy, and nightmares, and prevents memory loss and inefficiency. There are many chemotypes that have specific properties, including type linalol, which is not a skin irritant like the other thyme oils.

VANILLA (*Vanilla planifolia*)

The sweet, creamy scent—obtained with a resinoid, an absolute, an oleoresin, or by CO_2 extraction—improves lack of confidence and helps dissolve pent-up anger and frustration. It is consoling, and can unleash subconscious, hidden sensuality. Some psychoanalysts use it to bring back childhood memories.

VETIVER (*Vetiveria zizanoides*)

Distilled from root, the scent is earthy and heavy. Vetiver eases muscular pain, sprains, and liver congestion, and is a circulatory stimulant. Externally it treats acne, wounds, and dry skin. Vetiver is uplifting, relaxing, and comforting, releasing deep fears and tensions. It cools the body and mind of excessive heat. In India and Indonesia, door and window screens called "tatties," woven from the roots, are sprinkled with water on hot days to scent and cool the house. An inferior oil is made from the used screens.

YLANG-YLANG (*Cananga odorata*)

An intensely sweet, floral fragrance that some describe as banana-like is distilled from these tropical flowers. A strong sedative, ylang-ylang reduces muscle spasms and lowers blood pressure. As a hair tonic, it balances oil production. The fragrance makes the senses more acute and tempers depression, fear, jealousy, anger, and frustration. It is also an aphrodisiac, although high concentrations may produce headaches.

Glossary

Carbon dioxide extraction: CO_2 extraction is a new process that uses high pressure and low heat to extract essential oils. The fragrance is better preserved than with high-heat methods such as distillation, and CO_2 extraction leaves no solvent residue.

Carrier: Essential oils, to be used safely, almost always require dilution. The base in which they are diluted, usually vegetable oil or alcohol, is called a "carrier."

Chemotype: A term used by aromatherapy chemists to designate a plant that has a slightly different chemistry than others of the same species. These genetic variations are reproduced by cloning or cuttings, rather than by planting seeds. Different growing conditions will often produce a greater abundance of one or another chemotype group. Aromatherapists may seek out one chemotype because it is higher in a particular medicinal constituent.

Diffuser: This handblown glass apparatus pumps a consistent fine mist of unheated fragrance into the air. Because it operates on an electric pump, try to find one that doesn't make too much noise. Do not use thick oils such as vetiver, sandalwood, vanilla, myrrh, and benzoin in a diffuser unless they are diluted with thinner essential oils, or mixed with alcohol—otherwise, they may clog your diffuser. Also don't let essential oils sit for weeks in a diffuser. If your diffuser does get clogged, or if you just want to get rid of a permeating scent, rubbing alcohol is the best cleanser.

Distillation: A common method of extracting essential oils is by steam distillation. With this method, steam passing through the plant matter lifts the essential oil out of the plant. The oil-ladened steam is then forced into an enclosed condensation tube surrounded by a cold-water bath. The cold turns the steam back into water, separating out most essential oils into beads that may be skimmed off the surface of the water.

Enfleurage: This is probably the oldest method of extracting fragrance from plants. The fragrant part of the plant is placed on thin, warm layers of animal fat, which absorb the oil. Once the fat has been saturated with fragrance, the oil is separated out. Virtually obsolete today, enfleurage is still occasionally used for plants that are unable to withstand the intense heat of distillation. This method is especially appropriate for the flowers of jasmine or tuberose, which continue to manufacture essential oils after they are picked.

Fixative: Most essential oils slowly deteriorate with age (although some actually improve as they get older). Fixative oils are used by perfumers and other fragrance-makers so the finished product will smell better and last longer. Examples of fixative essential oils are clary sage, patchouli, sandalwood, vetiver, angelica, oakmoss, and most balsams, gums, and oleo-resins, such as benzoin, balsam of Peru, balsam of tolu, frankincense, myrrh, and styrax.

Fixed oil: Vegetable oils are called "fixed" because, unlike the molecules of essential oils, their molecules are too large to escape naturally from the plant. For the same reason, vegetable oils are not easily absorbed into the skin. Most vegetable oils are extracted by a combination of heat and pressure.

Fragrant water: Fragrant waters are produced by adding essential oils to distilled water. They are less expensive, but also less effective, moisturizing agents than hydrosols (see below). Spray or splash on a fragrant water after your shower, to cool down on a hot day or just to freshen your face.

Herb infusion: This is a fancy name for herb tea. Whenever you take a fragrant herb and steep it in boiling water, the essential oils are extracted into the water. You can also make an oil infusion by extracting essential oils from plants that are submerged in warm vegetable oil.

Hydrosol: The large amount of water used during steam distillation usually picks up some of the essential oil and, along with it, its fragrance. (This is especially true of an essential oil such as rose, which is partly water-soluble.) This by-product of distillation can be used in any application for which a water carrier is desired. The most popular uses of hydrosols are as facial sprays and as room spritzers. Hydrosols are impregnated with water-soluble ("hydrophilic") compounds that are not present in essential oils.

Volatile oil: Essential oils are sometimes called "volatile" because of how quickly they evaporate into the air and dissipate.

Dilutions and Doses

Bath: 3–15 drops in tub

Compress: 5 drops in 1 cup of water

Cream and lotion: stir in 3–6 drops for every ounce of cream or lotion

Douche: 3–5 drops in 1 quart of warm water

Facial clay: 3 drops in 1 tablespoon prepared clay (water already added)

Foot or hand bath: 5–10 drops for every quart of water

Fragrant water: 5–10 drops in 4 ounces of water

Gargle or mouthwash: 1–2 drops in 1/4 cup of water

Inhalant: 3–5 drops in bowl of hot water

Light bulb ring: 2–3 drops on ring

Liniment: 15–18 drops essential oil for every ounce of carrier oil

Massage/body oil: 10 drops essential oil for every ounce of carrier oil

Perfume: one drop for fragrance

Potpourri: 1/2 teaspoon essential oils to 2 cups dried herbs

Room spray: 20 drops per 4 ounces of water (shake before using)

Salve: stir in 12–24 drops per 2 ounces of salve

Sitz bath: 5–10 drops in basin large enough to sit in

Washes: 6–12 drops in small basin of water

Measurements

The following chart will help you through the maze of measurements used in aromatherapy. It will guide you to finding the proper measurements when you convert formulas. Most books indicate formulas by the drop, but some use teaspoons or milliliters instead. The chart will also help you to do price comparisons when you buy essential oils from different sources. This can get confusing because they are sold by the ounce, dram, or milliliter.

APPROXIMATE MEASUREMENT CONVERSION CHART

12 drops	1/8 tsp.	1/48 oz.	1/6 dram	5/8 ml.
25 drops	1/4 tsp.	1/24 oz.	1/3 dram	1-1/4 ml.
100 drops	1 tsp.	1/6 oz.	1-1/3 dram	5 ml.
150 drops	1-1/2 tsp.	1/4 oz.	2 drams	7.5 ml.
300 drops	1 T.	1/2 oz.	4 drams	15 ml.

24 tsp.	8 T.	4 oz.	1/2 cup	1/4 pint
48 tsp.	16 T.	8 oz.	1 cup	1/2 pint
96 tsp.	32 T.	16 oz.	2 cups	1 pint

The most common dilution for aromatherapy formulas is a 2 percent dilution, or 12 drops essential oil per ounce of carrier (vegetable oil, alcohol, or water).

Resources

Schools and Correspondence Courses

Victoria Edwards
Aromatherapy Institute and Research Center
P.O. Box 2354
Fair Oaks, CA 95628
Aromatherapy seminars

Mindy Green
c/o Rocky Mountain Center for Botanical Studies
P.O. Box 19254
Boulder, CO 80308-2254
Herb and aromatherapy classes and seminars

Kathi Keville
Oak Valley Herb Farm
P.O. Box 2482
Nevada City, CA 95959
Herb and aromatherapy classes and seminars

Dorene Petersen
Australasian College of Herbal Studies
P.O. Box 57
Lake Oswego, OR 97034
(800) 48-STUDY
Aromatherapy-certificate home study

Jeanne Rose
Aromatherapy Study Course
219 Carl St.
San Francisco, CA 94117
Correspondence course and seminars

Kurt Schnaubelt
The Aromatherapy Course
P.O. Box 66
San Rafael, CA 94903
Correspondence course and seminars

Michael Scholes
Aromatherapy Seminars
3370 South Robertson Blvd.
Los Angeles, CA 90034
(800) 677-2368
Correspondence course and seminars
Newsletter: *Beyond Scents*

Organizations and Newsletters

American Alliance of Aromatherapy
P.O. Box 750428
Petaluma, CA 94975-0428
(707) 769-5120
Newsletter: *News Quarterly*
Distributes: *International Journal of Aromatherapy*

American Herb Association
P.O. Box 1673
Nevada City, CA 95959
(916) 265-9552
Newsletter: *AHA Quarterly*
(includes herbs and aromatherapy)
Offers: *AHA Directory of Mail Order Herbal and Aromatherapy Products* ($4) and *AHA Directory of Herbal Education* (includes aromatherapy) ($3.50)

National Association for Holistic Aromatherapy
P.O. Box 17622
Boulder, CO 800308-0622
Newsletter: *Scentsitivity*

Canadian and English Associations

Association of Tisserand Aromatherapists
44 Ditchling Rise
Brighton, East Sussex BNI 3PY
England
Newsletter: *International Journal of Aromatherapy*

Canadian Federation of Aromatherapists
Box 68571-1235 Williams Pky. East
Brampton, Ontario L6S 6A1
Newsletter: *Escential News*

International Federation of Aromatherapists
46 Dalkeith Rd., Dulwich
London SE21 8LS
England

Mail Order Essential Oils and Products

Aroma Land
Rt. 20, P.O. Box 29AL
Santa Fe, NM 87505
(800) 933-5267
Aroma jewelry and lamps

Oak Valley Herb Farm
P.O. Box 2482
Nevada City, CA 95959
Essential oils, aromatherapy massage bath and body oils, cosmetics, herbal products; catalog $1

Original Swiss Aromatics
P.O. Box 606
San Rafael, CA
Essential oils, base ingredients, cosmetics; catalog $1

Prima Fleur Botanicals
1201-R Anderson Dr.
San Rafael, CA 94901
(415) 455-0956
Essential oils

Simpler's Botanical Co.
P.O. Box 39
Forestville, CA 95436
Hydrosols, essential oils, carrier oils, herbal extracts, cosmeticswelcome datacomp

Professional Associations and Journals

The Flavor and Extract Manufacturers'
Association of the United States (FEMA)
900 17th St. NW
Washington, DC 20006

Journal of Essential Oil Research
Allured Publishing Corporation
362 S Schmale Rd.
Carol Stream, IL 60188
(708) 653-2155

Perfumer and Flavorist (journal)
Allured Publishing Corporation
2100 Manchester Rd., Bldg. C, Suite 1600
Wheaton, IL 60187

U.S. Essential Oil Trade (1993 publication)
Circular Series
U.S. Department of Agriculture
Foreign Agricultural Service
Room 4655-S
Washington, DC 20250-1000

Essential Oils Distillers

Pope Scientific, Inc.
P.O. Box 495
Menominee Falls, WI 53052-0495
(414) 251-930

INDEX

Pocket Guides from The Crossing Press

To receive a current catalog from The Crossing Press
please call toll-free, 800-777-1048.
Visit our Web site: www. crossingpress.com